The Thief In The Night

My Journey through Acquired Brain Injury

Catherine
O'Toole Scott

chipmunkapublishing
the mental health publisher

Published by
Chipmunkapublishing
United Kingdom

http://www.chipmunkapublishing.com

ISBN 978-1-78382-203-4

Contents

Author's Note

It might be noted that aspects of my book might seem repetitive in places. This has caused something of an editorial dilemma because although to be editorially 'correct', the repetitions aren't really desirable; in truth my tendency for repetition is a symptom of my brain injury, which is what the book is about. My journals contain endless repetitions as I struggled to make sense of things around me and although many have been removed, some aspects of repetition have been retained, so that my book reflects as closely as possible my true experience of recovery.

On the subject of repetition and for additional clarity, readers may want to note that both my son and my son-in-law are named Simon.

Finally, I am sure there are many versions of how I was affected by Encephalitis and my subsequent journey to recovery. The Thief in the Night – My Journey through Acquired Brain Injury is my experience, my story and record of how and what happened to me. What I write does in no way detract from anybody else's version of my story.

I dedicate this book to all who have suffered from Encephalitis and to all the families and friends who have been affected by the devastation left in its wake, *especially my children and their families.*

Foreword

Last year I was writing a book review, something that I am often asked to do. I commented that the particular book, a memoir of the wife of a brain injury survivor, was *'a great addition to the brain injury literature'*. Having submitted my review it was suggested to me that such comment is probably best reserved for the academic literature, and I might like to substitute the wording. I disagreed then as I do now and resultantly did not change my choice of words. That book, like this book, *is* a valuable addition to the brain injury literature. In this case particularly to the literature around Encephalitis, about which little exists in reality.

Catherine's story is important. It is her narrative, and important for that alone, however it is important for a number of other reasons. It is an honest and candid account of her outcomes following Encephalitis and the impact it has had both upon her and her family. It will help others to feel better understood and less alone. It also demonstrates that the outcomes of Encephalitis, in those likely to be considered mildly or moderately affected in a clinical sense, can in fact find life on a day to day basis extremely difficult and at times hopeless. The labels we rely upon, and to some extent impose upon survivors of this devastating condition can, at times, serve only to confuse and perhaps dismiss their experiences.

We have called Encephalitis *'A Thief'* for many years at The Encephalitis Society. It robs people of abilities we take for granted every day: thinking, memory, concentration, inhibitions. For some families it robs them of their loved one and even in those families where the person affected survives, it can rob them of the person they once knew.

It is my pleasure to know Catherine both as a member of our Society and as one of our dedicated and highly valued regional volunteers. The ability to write is a gift and this book is a gift to the many survivors (and their family members and friends) who will read it and will feel someone *does* understand, and they are not so alone. I am conscious that the candid way in which this book and its contents have been presented will have left its mark upon Catherine. The process of writing for many people can of course be a therapeutic one and I am sure that its culmination and publication is all part of the recovery journey that forms the central theme of the book. It is an honour to have been asked to contribute this Foreword.

The Thief in the Night also has much to offer health, social care and education professionals who go on to support Encephalitis Survivors. I have been working in the field of Encephalitis now for over 15 years. I read many academic papers and they certainly add a great deal to our understanding. However my greatest learning has come from the stories of survivors and their families, and that is why this book is such a useful addition to the Encephalitis and brain injury literature.

Dr Ava Easton, PhD
Chief Executive
The Encephalitis Society

January 2015

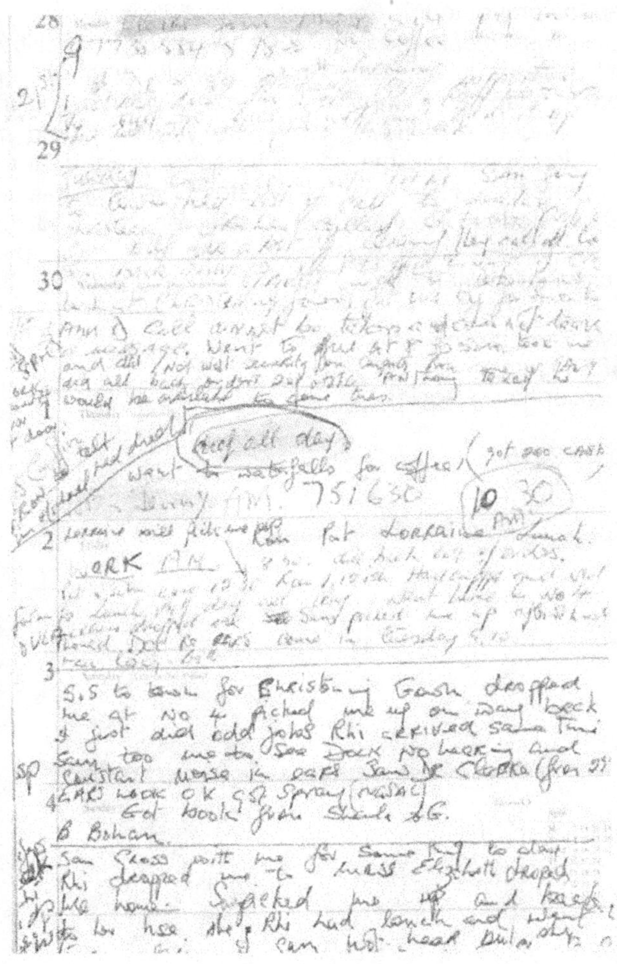

	Morning	Lunch	Tea	Bed
[illegible] – as required 4 hourly	7 ✓	✓	✓	✓
…acetamol x2 tablets – as required 4 hourly	7 ✓	2 PM ✓	✓	✓
…piclone – x1 tablet before bed				✓
TUESDAY	Morning	Lunch	Tea	Bed
…isolone	✓			
5mg Tablets – with or after food	7.30			
…eprazole Gastro Resistant x1 Tablet	7.30 ✓			
…ecalm x1 tablet – as required 4 hourly	7.30 ✓	✓	✓	✓
…acetamol x2 tablets – as required 4 hourly	7.30 ✓	✓	✓	✓
…piclone – x1 tablet before bed				✓
WEDNESDAY	Morning	Lunch	Tea	Bed
…isolone	✓			
5mg Tablets – with or after food	7.30			
…eprazole Gastro Resistant x1 Tablet	7.30 ✓			
…ecalm x1 tablet – as required 4 hourly	7.30 ✓	✓	✓	✓
…acetamol x2 tablets – as required 4 hourly	7AM	✓	✓	✓
…piclone – x1 tablet before bed				[illegible]
THURSDAY	Morning	Lunch	Tea	Bed
…isolone	✓			
5mg Tablets – with or after food	6.30			
…eprazole Gastro Resistant x1 Tablet	6.30 ✓			
…ecalm x1 tablet – as required 4 hourly	6.30 ✓	✓	✓	✓
…acetamol x2 tablets – as required 4 hourly	6.30 ✓	✓	✓	✓
…piclone – x1 tablet before bed				✓
FRIDAY	Morning	Lunch	Tea	Bed
…isolone	✓			
5mg Tablets – with or after food	7.30			
…eprazole Gastro Resistant x1 Tablet	7.30 ✓			
…ecalm x1 tablet – as required 4 hourly	7.30 ✓	✓	✓	✓
…acetamol x2 tablets – as required 4 hourly	7.30 ✓	✓	✓	✓
…piclone – x1 tablet before bed	[illegible]			✓
…dronic Acid – x1 tablet in the morning with water **…it for 30mins before taking any meds or food**	6.30 ✓			10.30
SATURDAY	Morning	Lunch	Tea	Bed
…isolone	✓			
5mg Tablets – with or after food	7.30			
…eprazole Gastro Resistant x1 Tablet	7.30 ✓			
…ecalm x1 tablet – as required 4 hourly	7.30 ✓	✓	✓	✓
…acetamol x2 tablets – as required 4 hourly	7.30 ✓	✓	✓	✓
…piclone – x1 tablet before bed				[illegible]
SUNDAY	Morning	Lunch	Tea	Bed
…isolone	✓			
5mg Tablets – with or after food	7.30			
…eprazole Gastro Resistant x1 Tablet	7.30 ✓			
…ecalm x1 tablet – as required 4 hourly	7.30 ✓	✓	✓	✓
…acetamol x2 tablets – as required 4 hourly	7.30 ✓	✓	✓	✓
…piclone – x1 tablet before bed				✓

Paracetamol AM only x

Catherine O'Toole Scott

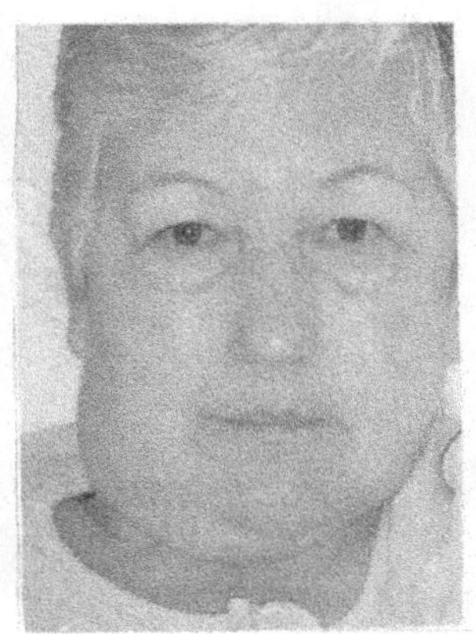

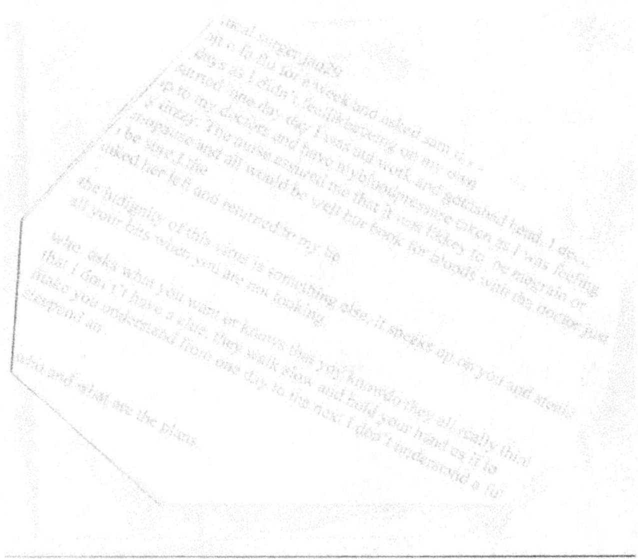

ical surgery jan29
on a flu for a week and asked sam u...
days as I didn't feellikebeeing on my own
started one day day I was aat work and gotaslied head. I de...
up to my doctors and have myblood pressure taken as I was feeling
y dizzy. The nurse assured me that it was likley to be megrain or
menopause and all would be well but book for bloods with the doctor just
to be sure I the
thanked her left and returned to my be

the indignity of this virus is something else, it sneeks up on you and steals
all your bits when you are not looking.

who asks what you want or knows that you know do they all really thin
that I don't have a clue, they walk slow and hold your hand as if to
make you understand from one day to the next I don't understand a fu
steppend on.

who and what are the plans.

Introduction

You never know what's around the corner, yet I'm someone who's always been pretty happy with that kind of unpredictability - it suits my nature for life to throw up surprises for me to explore. In truth, I secretly relish investigating new things, because these hold the potential for both educating as well as challenging me. Of course, I'm not always successful in my endeavours, but I hold dear what I learn in the process.

Over the years, what some would see as fortitude, others a keenness to make something of myself, and a few more as downright stubbornness, my willingness to explore opportunities thrown up by the quirks of life has served me in good stead: twists in the course of 'true love' which left me divorced with two young children became a quest to earn enough to look after them independently; being made redundant twice from private companies supplying the health service left me to pursue financial security once again, this time in the form of partnering up with a colleague to run our own business which made the most of our experience. Squaring up to this as both an opportunity and a challenge, we built a business specialising in bespoke seating and postural control for the severely disabled. Ahh yes, the irony! And when my business partner retired? I was happy to take the reins myself and pursue my own course as a totally independent business woman.

Something was still missing though. Although my role was fulfilling, working in an industry serving the special needs sector wasn't quite enough, didn't really seem to give enough back. So, always one to add another string to my bow, I studied and qualified as a professional counsellor too, working at my local counselling service – all aspects of my professional life poised to assist others, whatever position they find themselves in within their own.

Meanwhile, my children, my daughter and son, grew into adults. My son returned to my native Ireland to live and work and my daughter, now married, lived by the seaside. From her vantage point of the South coast, life seemed pretty good, so it wasn't long before I relocated my business and my home down to the seaside too, a timely move as soon afterwards, when I was fifty seven, came the announcement of my daughter's expectation of a whole new generation for our family.

Now I know fifty seven might seem pretty old in terms of many families, but at that time I didn't think of myself as a potential grandparent and I still don't see myself as being of that generation - somehow, that seems to be a role for parents older than myself. My own connotations of what it means to be a grandparent, what it means to be "old" - in the generational sense, as much as the passing of years and physical aging process - won't let me believe that I'm really there, or at least they didn't.

In the wake of an unwelcome virus, a thief in the night, I find myself denoted as a family elder in all senses of the word. Yet whilst people constantly want to compare my incapacity with what happens as we age, they are missing a vital point; I did not get the opportunity to age with any grace or dignity, it happened almost overnight.

"I tell you solemnly, anyone who does not enter the sheepfold through the gate, but gets in by some other way is a thief and a brigand."

John 10: 1 - 10

1. A Long Day's Work

The diary's already filling up fast and we haven't even got to the end of January yet! Both aspects of my work are extremely busy and, whether I'm at the counselling service or in my own office, I find myself still playing catch-up from those Christmas and New Year breaks. Well, that and covering for those off sick with seasonal ills. I always think myself lucky to avoid these and this winter I'm doing pretty well in avoiding the sniffles which have been unrelenting across both offices and all their respective clients. Apart from a real cold spell back in December, they say it's been slightly warmer than usual so far this winter. Mind you, this January weather remains relentlessly wet, like it's been raining forever; great weather for ducks - and germs.

That said, and despite the fact I'm quite glad to be back in the routine, it's only 17th of January and I'm starting to feel the strain of it all a little more than usual. Maybe it's because things are so busy? Perhaps it's the persistence of the rain? It certainly feels like it's all a bit much today. As I look around the counselling service office, with its sticky-tack pocked walls marking the spots of the recently departed festive cheer, I feel there's nothing like being in this hub of professional positivity, draped in its January drear, to give you the blues.

But no, this feeling's more than about being here, today ... it really feels more like that post-Christmas "I really want a holiday in the sun" feeling. My family and I have been making plans to head off this mood since long before Advent though, planning ahead to make the most of the time left of Sam's maternity leave with a holiday for all of us - Sam and Simon, baby Evie, Simon's mother and me! That's all booked and now, more than ever, I'm really looking forward to it.

So no, with my holiday to look forward to I haven't really got the blues either, I decide as I squint at my papers and try to feel purposeful. This heavy feeling isn't emotional, it's physical. The truth is, I don't actually feel too good and I'm more than a little dizzy. The papers seem to swim in front of me, it's just like trying to look through the rain-splashed window and there's a dull, repetitive thud emanating from some point in my heavy head.

Oh no, not again, surely? I shut my eyes against the pain and recall my trip to London, just before Christmas, to the glitzy AGM and new design awards celebration for the trade association I belong to, for my postural control and special seating business. As usual, I'd looked forward to attending, going about my usual routine of planning and preparation with something pretty close to excitement. I'd booked a hotel close to the venue, taking care to choose a good one, because I do love staying in a good hotel and enjoying all the extras like the large baths and luxury toiletries, making the most of the away-from-home treats. I'd also relished the annual thrill of picking out a suitable dress - in keeping with both the occasion and my role in business, but also for myself, as a woman – this gathering's my one chance a year to indulge myself in buying something special. The right dress is important for many reasons, not least because it's a black-tie, dressy do with good company and superb food, but because I spend the year working hard, flitting between my business and my counselling job and I deserve this end-of-year frivolity!

So I'd looked forward to it as usual and even more so because it was being held at the Central Hall, Westminster, where we were accompanied by our parliamentary advisor and where the elegant and admirable Angela Rippon was presiding over the proceedings. Yet although I wore my new dress and joined my colleagues in most of the festivities, as the late night slid into early morning I began to feel the need for more fresh air breaks. I started to remove myself to the crispy leaf-covered street, watching the rest of the city passing and crunching winter underfoot, not because I was hot, but to seek a fresh-air remedy for what seemed to be the start of a headache although not, it seemed, a headache borne of the bubbling champagne, the eloquently enthusiastic Ms. Rippon or the noisy, happy party. This was much more an insidious kind of headache, with a sinister, sickly approach which, despite the joy in my surroundings and the company, brought with it a companion of inexplicable nervousness.

In the end, when the December fresh air gave up being helpful but turned instead into the risk of hypothermia,

I had retreated, making a quiet exit, long before the event was due to finish. I had hailed a taxi back to my hotel and, ignoring the allure of the long hot bath of treats I'd promised myself, I just crawled into bed to get my self-destructing head onto the comfort of a pillow. I don't remember much more about it, except as I'd closed my eyes I remember thinking, please God, don't let me die here!

I shudder as I recall the pain and loneliness of that night. If I could shake my head at myself without it hurting then I would do ... surely that was just a one-off, a migraine? Apparently not a one-off though, as today another seems to be building. It's probably my blood pressure again. Although being fifty seven and not having high blood pressure is a bonus for heart-health, being prone to low blood pressure isn't a barrel of laughs as an alternative. I decide to head-off this headache and the possibility of another awful migraine by getting my blood pressure checked.

Decision made, I'm gentle with myself as I abandon my papers and get up, making sure not to exacerbate my symptoms by standing up too quickly. I wander over to Dave's desk. He's a good manager, always thinks of the person, so he's affable about me popping out to the doctor's and tells me to take care of myself. He's a counsellor alright.

I'm patting my coat pockets down for my car keys for a good minute before I remember that I didn't bring the car today. This is what I get for wanting to take the healthy advantage of walking from home to the counselling centre - I've left myself feeling grotty and stranded. A walk to the surgery from here is just a walk too far in this miserable weather so, feeling pretty annoyed with myself, I book a taxi. This isn't a decision I take lightly - the distance to the surgery will clock up several pounds on the taxi's meter, but a ghostly shadow of creeping nervousness from that night in London is sending shivers through me, so I don't feel I have any choice; something more than the pressure in my skull is pushing me to check in with the doctor.

#

Of course, it's never as easy as that. Despite the cost of the taxi, I'm not able to see the doctor, thanks to the wonders of the strict appointments system and the even stricter receptionist. Instead, I sit, immersed in the steaming soup of germs in the waiting room, trying to keep my eyes closed against the worst of the overhead, fluorescent glare, until the nurse is able to see me.

"Your blood pressure's fine," she reassures me, as she removes the pressure cuff and I begin to tug my sleeve back down my arm. "Your headache's most likely caused by the menopause, or it's just a migraine."

We exchange that look, the universal one which passes between women of a certain age every time the menopause is mentioned. She smiles and continues brightly as she turns to her computer.

"Best to double check things though. Can you pop back in on Monday and I'll take some bloods?"

I agree the appointment and drag my weary body and hormone head home.

#

The bloods appointment comes and goes, but it's not the highlight of the week for me. I still feel dreadful. There's no really a list of symptoms, apart from this headache, but I'm so dragged down by this off-colour feeling and it's been such a long time since I've visited the GP that, in truth, I'm not altogether comfortable about the diagnosis. I decide I need to see Dr. Shen, my Chinese herbalist, back up in Sutton. She says she can fit me in for the coming Friday, January 24th, which seems ideal. I have some counselling workshops on the Saturday, but then I can take the remainder of the weekend to rest and allow the acupuncture and any herbs she gives me to do their work. I'm inordinately reassured as I write the appointment carefully down in my diary and for the rest of the week I work towards this day with a sense of impending relief, oblivious to the fact that in its shadow, follows terror.

#

Friday 24th arrives. Despite still feeling weighed down by my own head and a warning weariness in my limbs, I manage to get myself on the right train to Sutton, in plenty of time for my appointment. The rhythm of the train alternates disconcertingly between offerings of a soothing lull or piercing screech to my head, so I try to distract myself with positive thinking about the appointment, whilst not catching the eye of other travellers. Normally I'd chat to anyone to pass the time but not today; I don't have a conversation in me.

Instead, I consider with confidence the help the train is rushing me towards. After all, my herbalist is a professor, an absolute specialist in her field, upon whom I've totally relied for many years. She's always been spot on with her diagnoses and treatments and we've come to know each other well. Ironically, given the nurse's mention of the big M, I actually found Dr. Shen's clinic when my original menopausal symptoms started to develop, way back in 1997.

I'd had blood tests with my GP at the time who, after first helpfully suggesting that I might have glandular fever, eventually wanted to prescribe the middle-aged dread that comes hand-in-hand with middle-aged-spread and hormone head: HRT, hormone replacement treatment. So of course, like a good patient, I'd gone along with the idea and put up with it for a few months but it didn't actually take that long for me to realise that it really didn't suit me at all. In return for my dedication to the medication, I just piled on weight and felt no better than I did before. In fact, if anything, I was more miserable.

One day at work, after exploring the issue within the gentle camaraderie of exchanged confidences and shared concern from female work colleagues at the time, I'd declared: "I just can't go on like this, I have to find another way."

My colleagues responded magnificently to the call to action with a collective uptake of local phone books, as there was of course no Google in our office back then. In a joint effort, we looked up all the complementary therapists in a reasonable distance from either my home or the office. By chance or intervention, somehow we settled on an herbalist's number. I still can't explain why I felt drawn to it but, mystical forces aside, practicalities made her the first and most logical choice: her practice was in Sutton, wonderfully accessible to me as I would pass it on my way to and from home on an office day. When I rang she gave me an appointment for that afternoon and that's where the relationship began.

Dr. Shen is highly qualified and always works in conjunction with people's prescribed medicines; indeed, she has an amazing knowledge of conventional medicine and has been on the NHS advisory board for Chinese Herbal

Medicine. What's more, from a patient's perspective, she's wonderful, offering timely advice as well as intervention and expert, effective acupuncture and treatment. After so many years of treating me, she knows me well - particularly my pulse and body - and for my part I trust her professional opinion implicitly. We've also had many laughs in our communications as she has tried to understand my broad western Irish accent and I've struggled with her soothing Chinese cadence. In pursuit of clarity, we often end up in the throes of hilarity as we use diagrams of body parts, plants, herbs and on one bizarre occasion even meat cuts to try to ensure we properly understand each other!

On this visit, I arrive at the clinic in Sutton in something of a heap of fatigue. Dr. Shen greets me with a warm, but concerned expression and, once I'm settled, she takes my pulse, as usual. I almost want her to just put her hand on my head, like a mother, to make it all go away but as a consummate professional she does the next best thing - she tells me that I have a virus invading my body and offers me an acupuncture session, which I gratefully accept. However, something's missing from our usual interactions. Try as I might, I just can't concentrate or hold onto her words today. I lie on the couch, preparing for her needles, trying to recall what she just said is wrong with me. I draw a blank and try again but I might as well try to retrace my steps in sinking sand for all the good thinking about it does me, her words are lost. As I realise this I find, with a sense of some comfort, that it doesn't really matter; I neither know nor even care what's going on or whether the treatment is curative or preventative … I just want relief, in whatever form, from my own head.

The session passes in a blur of needle-pricks and relaxation which seem to exhaust me. Seemingly moments later, although it's been over an hour, I find myself making my way to the clinic exit, carrying a month's worth of herbs, which I'm told will protect my brain from the virus. As I leave, the professor continues to give me instructions, her face earnest with concern. Whatever else I don't understand about today, she's adamant that I need to be taking these herbs, that much I do grasp.

I try to concentrate on making my way safely back to Sutton Station, where I double-check platform numbers and the train times which dance alarmingly across the screens as I struggle to ensure that I can at least get onto the right train. This part of the plan my mind and body are just about in agreement over - not only the need to get home safely, but also to not have to think again until I arrive back in St. Leonard's.

I stand, with a spiteful, splitting head, on the chilly platform, waiting for the train. I'm trying to concentrate on the instructions I've only just been given, but the words seem to have slipped away, somewhere just out of my grasp. The elusiveness of such essential information starts to frighten me. I try to think calmly, whilst my brain seems hell-bent on tap dancing in my head, but it's no use, once more I've lost the professor's vital words. I fumble with my mobile and phone Sam, partly to let her know I'm on my way back and partly to check that I still have words of my own. Although I do manage to speak to her, it seems I'm no more capable of a sensible conversation now than I was on the way up, so we speak for just moments before I hang up. My head feels massive, as if my brain is expanding beyond the confines of my skull, a great sense of pressure needing release.

Into the mix comes again that strange, sense of deja-vue. I'm disembodied as my sensibilities return me again to that hotel room in London, on the night of the AGM. The same pressure in my head, the same encompassing fear that I might not get through the night, except this time all I want to do is to be able to get home. A fear, similar to that night, is building. Raw and instinctive, it's not a fear borne of rationalities or of what ifs, in fact I have no sense of what might happen *if* ... if I don't manage to get on the train, if I don't get home, if I pass out ... I have no headspace to think about that, there's just a nothingness caught up in a grasping terror somewhere in my chest and the blanket of pressure in my skull which seems to be wrapped tight around one thought and one thought only: please God, let me make this journey home.

#

It's the next day and I'm not myself. In contrast to yesterday's heaviness I feel strangely light-headed, lost. And somewhere, in this mist of light, is the last twenty-four hours. I struggle through my day at the counselling service's Cognitive Behavioural Therapy (CBT) workshops, trying to be attentive but also trying to recall my journey home yesterday. I have some vague recall of putting the herbs to soak, an auto-pilot response to my visit to Dr. Shen, having done this for ten years or more. The intention is to boil them later, I'm sure. Yes, I must remember to boil them later, I think, when I get home.

At the end of the workshops, my colleagues seem to be making an unnecessary clamour with their cheery going-home routines whilst I quietly try to fathom my next move. Fear and weariness arrive once more like unwelcome guests as I struggle into my coat and I know I don't want to go home. Out comes my mobile and I fumble around, trying to access Sam's number in my contacts. It seems to be bizarrely difficult, yet appeals to me as an infinitely easier option than trying to remember her number and focus my finger onto each individual, fidgety digit.

"Sam, I don't feel very well," I mumble as she picks up the call. "Can I come to yours tonight?" The words are out of my mouth before I realise that this is what I'm thinking, what I want. I'm not sure why I should want to go to Sam's, I'm perfectly capable of being sick on my own, but somehow my words escape, revealing a need I didn't even know was there. As she agrees, I'm too tired to be effusive with my thanks, but I know I am thankful because gratitude and relief arrive instantly and start to elbow away some of this inexplicable fear.

#

I'm in my bed at Sam's house. At least, I think it's Sam's - it's not mine. How did I get here? I seem to remember driving my car, yet I can see myself, waiting in the doorway of the training venue because Sam's insisted on picking me up. The image of joining them for dinner swims past me ... that seems right; I ate dinner with them but just wanted to lay my head down, up here in the bed. But how did I get here? Why am I so tired?

#

This bed hurts me. It's hot and the sheets are wet, nasty. I feel the rivulets of sweat running down my legs, face, between my breasts as I'm blistered by sheets which stick vengefully to me, liquid and scorching. Am I in a hot bath? How can this really be a bed? It doesn't smell like a sweaty bed, the summer kind. This bed scorches and smells differently, a stench of sickness.

#

I'm trying to sleep but the noise disturbs me. Someone's moaning and groaning, I hear it in my wakeful moments. I'm surrounded by the sounds and smells of sickness, which just won't leave me be, just won't let me sleep.

#

"It's a migraine, I'll prescribe you some co-codamol" the out-of-hours doctor barely looks up. I'm up and about, shaky and still raging in my head but cooler in my body. I can't take co-codamol, it makes me sick. I know this but somehow I don't think to say it. I don't say much to him, really, I'm too tired. If Sam hadn't insisted on seeing the doctor, I'd still be in my bed. As it is, we've had to come all the way up here, to the out of hours Seadoc service at the hospital. I'm here at the hospital where, ironically, I feel far too ill to be ... all I want to do is get back to bed.

#

Ceiling views, bucket views, little else for two days. I roll in the bed, head still screaming, body now heaving with the inevitable vomiting from the medication. My own GP appears and I'm grateful for her needle, as effective as acupuncture but of course pharmaceutically laced to stop the vomiting. Paracetamol only, for the head and fever, from now on.

#

It's Thursday January 29th and I'm out of bed again, feeling a little better in both my head and body; today there seems to be some sort of unity between the two of them. Shakily, I manage a shower. Although it's not my preferred cleansing routine, it's both efficient and sufficient for removing the stench of illness that seems to be trailing after me like ... well, like a bad smell. It's a relief to get rid of it.

Even after the exertions of the shower, I don't actually feel too bad in myself. Sam kindly reminds me that I have a hairdresser's appointment and I decide I'm going to keep it. I'm already fed up with being sick and getting my hair sorted will do me good. I build a plan around this idea.

My office is on the way, so I decide I should try to pop into work, my company, for an hour before the appointment.

As the idea occurs I realise with something of a shock that I seem to have given little thought to work, either my company or the counselling service, for almost a week. This isn't like me … I'm usually so aware, so on top of my responsibilities, yet here I am, forgetting that I even have any. I try to set myself straight, but immediately struggle to think what today's responsibilities might be. There are invoices to be done, I'm sure. That would be both a useful task to do and an easy one for easing me back into work. After all, invoicing is a routine task for me, it takes an hour, tops.

The staff are glad to see me and after their effusive well-wishing and updating of news which I can't really take in, still tired I guess, I retreat to the comforting thought of doing something productive with those invoices. The trouble is, that's kind of only how far I get: retreating with them; thinking about them. I don't seem to be able to get through them, at least nothing like my usual number and, to tell the truth, I don't feel confident about what I'm doing. I'm conscious of trying to carry on as usual in front of my staff whilst I scrutinize the numbers with amazement and bewilderment. Dates, quantities, costs, measurements … so many numbers! They're usually meaningful and friendly to me, to the company, they show me the trade we're doing and how successfully things are working out. But today they're not my friends. Today they seem an ugly, unruly crowd, they're jostling in my head and all shouting so much, making so much noise that each and every one is meaningless and overwhelming.

Exasperated, I call it a day before the hour is up and wander off instead to keep my hair appointment. I chit chat with the hairdresser who's equally sympathetic to my recent indisposition, but really the chat is all hers. I'm just having a cut but I might just as well be wearing the little rubber cap for old-style highlights for the way her conversation bounces off me, meaningless and, literally, over my head. At my best, I know I'm usually much more attentive and responsive than this and even on an off-day I'd normally at least I'd make an effort to engage … but today? I try to chat but it's not even half-hearted really. Maybe I'm not quite as well yet as I thought?

I get a cab back to Sam's, grateful to rest in the back whilst the driver just transports me. Sam greets me warmly, glad to see that I've managed my tasks of the day. She tells me that she needs to pop to the supermarket so she can get some bits for dinner and invites me to join her, which of course I'm happy to do, I can always have a rest afterwards, can't I?

As we wander the aisles, a couple of magazines catch my eye. Perhaps I should indulge myself, have a feet-up evening with some gentle reading? I choose a couple and pop them into my basket. When I look up, I notice Sam's looking at me rather quizzically.

"You're buying those?"

I mistake her question for critical review. "Ah, they're fine ... I don't want anything too heavy going, you know, with the migraines?"

She shakes her head. "No, Mum, I mean, how are you buying those? Where's your handbag?"

"Ah, it's at your house."

"Well, how are going to pay for your shopping then?"

Somehow, I don't even need to pause to think of the answer. "It's OK, you can pay for them."

She continues to stare at me. It's possible she thinks I'm joking, but to me the answer seems very simple and logical and I guess she thinks so too, because she pays for them and puts them in a carrier bag for me.

#

We're back at Sam's house. I relax for a while and play with baby Evie whilst Sam prepares the dinner and chats to her husband. I feel bad not doing my normal thing of being the one to help out, so I offer my assistance.

"Yes, could you lay the table, please?"

I open the cutlery drawer and reach in for the implements I need, taking out a handful and turning to the table to lay them out.

"Mum?"

"U-huh?"

Sam casts her eye pointedly over the table and then seems to be looking at me warily. "Mum, we're going to need more than dessert spoons, don't you think?"

I'm not entirely sure what she means, but she hands me other cutlery from the drawer and I put it carefully around the placemats, feeling a little chastised, but not really sure why, or what for. When I look up from the table, Sam is whispering to her husband, Simon, as she dishes up the food. We sit together to eat and, unsure whether I actually feel hungry or not, I make a start on my dinner. Sam offers to fill my water glass, but I don't really fancy it so I decline and carry on with my meal whilst their gentle chatter continues in the background, like a radio play.

Before long, it seems I am actually thirsty, even though I didn't think so before. Maybe it's the food, I need a little something to wash it down with. I reach for a nearby glass, which is now filled with water, drink from it, then replace it.

"Mum! What are you doing?" Sam seems horrified that I'm having a drink. Perhaps I shouldn't have said "no" before? I'm confused.

"That's Simon's glass, Mum ... you've just reached over and taken Simon's glass." Her tone is still incredulous but her eyes worried. She glances towards Simon and then back towards me.

"Mum ..." her voice now more concerned than surprised. "Mum, I think you need to see a doctor again, you don't seem yourself."

I look from one to the other of them, then back to the offending water glass. I can't really see what they mean about the glass, about not being myself, but I'm guessing they're right. I don't really need to think about it, much less disagree over it which might have been my usual course of action. It's surprising really, for years I've adamantly preferred my alternative remedies to medical intervention, but I trot out "OK, whatever you think" readily, happily, even.

Sam phones the out-of-hours service, whilst Simon and I remain quietly at the table. Piecing the conversation together from hearing one side only is easy enough, although I can't really seem to relate it to being myself she's talking about, as I grasp snatches of her concerned voice: "ill for the week ..." pause; "no, she's not behaving in her normal way, you know, she's really not herself ..." pause; "... couldn't pay for her shopping, that's not like her at all, she's the kind of person who offers to pay for *my* shopping..."

pause; "laid the table ... dessert spoons ..." pause; "I'd really like someone to take a look at her" pause; then lots of repeated "no" and "no, not at all." Eventually, after a slightly extended pause, the phone clicks off and Sam reappears back at the dining table.

"Alright?" Simon enquires.

"Yes, yes ... the doctor's coming," Sam shrugs and shakes her head. "Strange though," she comments, with a look of surprise, "they seemed more concerned about whether Mum's endangering us!" She nods towards me, "they asked me if you were being violent, or if you're hurting yourself ... if we needed the police?"

Simon shakes his head, seemingly also baffled by this but I don't react, can't react. In truth I don't really understand any of it, so it seems I can only share her bewilderment by personifying it.

#

The doctor is here, someone I've never met before or if I have, I don't recall. The usual, basic medical necessities of temperature and blood pressure are dealt with first, followed by a few physical investigations. He asks me to push against his hands with my own, then it's onto the sofa so that I can use my feet to push against him that way too. I don't feel much, except compliant, like a toddler doing as I'm told.

Then the examination moves into Master Mind mode. The doctor starts to ask me all kinds of questions. What's the Queen's name? Who's the Prime Minister? His questions are endless and not just tiresome, but silly. I can't help but think this. Why would you ask someone who's not herself who other people are? In truth, I don't really know who these people are he's asking about, but I have an answer for each of his questions, the first answer which springs to mind. The thing I'm not sure about is where in my mind the answers are coming from, it seems to be from the place with the same sense of "correct" spontaneity as the one which apparently inspired me to drink from my son-in-law's glass.

The session's lasting forever and I'm feeling tired. It doesn't really bother me whether the doctor can see this or not, I'm just at the point where I'd like it to stop. He decides that I need to be admitted into hospital and goes off to use the phone. Sam and Simon are looking at me. I don't know what they're expecting, in truth I don't actually know what I'm expecting, but I accept the doctor's suggestion - it's all OK with me.

Even as I'm watching them, to find out what I'm supposed to do next, things change and I don't spot how it happens. The doctor's no longer on the phone, it's Sam on the phone now and I'm supposed to be getting my shoes on. I don't feel confused by this, on the contrary, I feel remarkably affable and comfortingly detached, absolved of responsibilities - all I have to do is what I am told to do. As positions and people around me change, so too do my surroundings. I'm in Sam's house, now I'm outside, I'm in a car, now I'm at the hospital. I know this is the hospital because I know the door, I've seen the foyer before. I know where I am, even if I'm not really sure why I'm here. I'm not confused, scared or even in pain. I'm just tired, it's been a long day, like a long day's work. I'm just going to shut my eyes for a minute ...

2. Quiet Please, Thief at Work

Apparently I am in the hospital, ensconced in the Medical Admissions Unit. The truth is, I am largely oblivious to this fact. I lay here, the weight of my limbs pinning me to the bed, whilst the professionals around me go about their perfunctory, impersonal business of tests, in order to diagnose and then hopefully to treat me, their patient, the sleeping stranger. That's fair enough of course; I am a stranger to them. The main concern though is that I also appear to be a complete stranger to my family and, bizarrely, to myself. My detachment from both my surroundings and my companions is made complete by three things: apparent 'absences', an absolute confusion and an overwhelming fatigue.

So, for the most part, I sleep. This is an actual state of sleeping, not unconsciousness. They say I am not *un*conscious yet I know I am not the opposite: I am not conscious in the sense of having any kind of awareness – including being aware of either the place or the people who make up my surroundings. My daughter is eerily familiar; I recognise her, yet there's a man at my bedside to whom I have to be formally introduced. In the history of awkward introductions, this turns out to be a pretty big one. "It's Simon, mum ... I'm Simon, your son."

My ability to be a stranger knows no bounds. I'm oblivious to facts that the normal "me" would have known: that's my child, he's travelled directly from Ireland in response to the distress signal from his sister, he's here because he's worried about me, they all are ... bless them, God, help them. But no, instead of receiving his mother's gratitude or reassurance, this man they call my own son receives the blank stare and mono-syllabic communications of a stranger. He is yet another face in the sea of unrecognisable features which float around the bed whilst I bob along on waves of absence, fatigue, pain and drowsiness. Sometimes he's there, sometimes he's not ... or is it sometimes I'm here, and then again, I'm not?

#

The nurses swarm my bed, as purposeful and irritating as ants. Appliances are attached and then detached at regular intervals, syringes slipped into waiting veins, fluids removed and passed along to the jigsaw of departments who test, diagnose and bring the picture of a patient together. Microscopic dots of my bodily fluids are couriered to London and heaven knows where else – all in a day's work for the courier, a life possibly on the line for my panicking family. The nurse promises my family that the doctor will have a word. He does. The word is "unsure."

#

Test after test comes back clear – it's apparently good news, this elimination of many dire diagnoses.

The doctor tells my daughter. "Academically your mother is not ill; in fact she is quite healthy!"

However, at any given time I am either too absent, too asleep or too ill, to know how apparently healthy I am. I embody a home which boasts a timer switch to keep the lights on. I have the appearance of being lived-in whilst the owner's far, far away. This contradictory appearance is of course any passing thief's best ally. The light is on and all's well to the onlooker, yet the thief is inside, stripping away all that is most precious. This is what's happening; I lie here, inert, surrounded by others, being academically "healthy" whilst my body is ransacked by a thief, as yet unidentified.

I sleep through the continuing routines of the ward, including visiting times. My daughter is here, Sam, with her little girl. I seem to know that this is her little girl, but I don't know her name. It's not that I can't recall it – I don't feel that it's a tip-of-my-tongue away, I feel I just don't *know* it. But despite this I'm aware, with a sense that's caught between the spiritual and the physical, which I guess means it's actually instinct ... that this tiny little mite is part of me.

The identification of Sam as my daughter logically defines this charming, babe-in-arms as my grand-daughter. Yet simple facts about her, like her name, are locked somewhere inside me, a place inside that doesn't seem to function or at least doesn't allow me access. I call her "little baby girl." According to those around me, the man holding her is my son-in-law. I'm not sure what to do with this information – certainly not process, use or retain it. The clear implication that I'm supposed to know these things worries me. Yet, even as a fear about this absence of my own wisdom creeps into my core, so too does the blissful ignorance of more sleep.

#

I start to synchronise a little within the daily routines of the ward, the routines of the body. Even in this haze of blessed slumber, not unconscious but not awake, there are those most basic human levels of function to which my body seems to adhere – sleep and elimination. At times, I'm awake enough to respond to the wet, clenching gripe somewhere in my abdomen. On legs which don't seem to belong to me, I get out of bed, senses and the room both reeling, but unfortunately not in the same direction. My need is urgent and I set off, one foot shuffling beside the other on a floor which seems to bounce, even though I have no idea where I am or where I intend going - in all senses of that word. Someone walks me to the lavatory and, upon returning to my bed, I continue to sleep.

#

This ability to get up and function is deemed to be "A Good Thing", even though my awareness of it is limited to those personal performances which are a basic necessity. Showering, of course, is considered to be another of these. I shouldn't need telling of course; as 'me', I am the woman whom you can tell everything about by the contents of her handbag – a business woman, an independent woman, a well-groomed woman and mother, that's me, that's the kind of woman I am. Yet I seem to have been misplaced. Somehow, whilst the thief runs unchecked through the cranial crevices of my "self", the precious gems of my treasured memories, the charms of my character and even my crystal clarity of function are embezzled away; all that's left in this hospital bed is this stranger who might be me; this patient with the blank stare; this patient who has to be railroaded, upon white, shaking legs, to the shower.

My daughter takes me to the wet room. In the same instance when I realise that a shower would be acceptable, I also grasp that something which is totally unacceptable, to both aspects of 'me', is about to happen: I have to shower in front of my daughter. At some level of my confused processing, I understand this, yet at the same time I can't comprehend it. The presence of the only person who isn't a stranger to me, at the time when I'd most prefer a stranger? I need help, this I know, but my daughter? Why can't it be a nurse, someone who doesn't have an association with me, that physical link with the intimacies of this badly behaved body? Yet I don't have the words, ability or energy to object; I am a business woman, an independent woman, a proud woman, yet I take my showers whilst slumped on a chair in a sterile tiled cell, in my daughter's presence. Mortified does not even begin to cover it.

I lose days this way, trapped between the institutional routines of the hospital, the increasing detachment of my brain from my "self" and my "self" from my surroundings, all in a largely on-going slumber and distinct absences which seem to deteriorate, rather than restore, my health. My observations, both semi-lucid and completely fuddled don't take the form of eerie, ethereal out-of-body experiences you read about in those sensationalist "It Happened To Me!" articles. Instead I'm trapped in a series of brutal, blunt occurrences where my own vitality has been stolen away, from which, in the worst of all ironies, that stealthy insidious oblivion is my only respite.

These absences are as indefinable as they are indiscriminate. In contrast to the healing bliss of sleep or the protective ignorance of unconsciousness, my absences are a huge weight of nothingness. There's no poetic sensation of peering into a void: that would imply some kind of pro-activity or awareness on my own part. Instead, there's a pervading sense of nothing, the hypnotic monochrome of a cine film left running beyond its own very last moments. Possibly these are my own very last moments. I'm not just absent, I am empty. Gone.

#

This continued absence, interspersed with an all-encompassing exhaustion, serves only to add to my children's panic. We are inversions: I lie prone, lifeless and undemanding in the bed whilst they hover, pace and demand answers. Worn down with fear and frustration, they wait out that hideous hiatus from everyday normality that family traumas bring by clamouring to find out just what the hell is wrong with me. They want a diagnosis, not too much to ask and from there they want treatment, which is understandable. Then, after all that, they want their mum back, please – another very reasonable request. In conversations between themselves, the medical profession, God and the Saints, a pair of visiting nuns and practically any one else who might listen, my children repeatedly advocate on my behalf for these things. In return, I offer up my own subconscious prayer, that I might get better or die, whichever should come the soonest.

My daughter, as forthright as a lioness protecting its cub, demands more action, more scans. As a result, sometimes my surroundings alter. OK, so one hospital ceiling does look pretty much like another, but you know when you're on a trolley and moving along a corridor because, for a change, the morphing and movement of the ceiling isn't actually in your head. Instead it's because you're progressing at speed to the MRI facility for another scan, courtesy of either type of porter – the man-of-few-words type, or the chirpy chappy whose mum had this done and it's no bother at all.

He's right of course, the chirpy chappy, it is no bother. It's neither painful nor even uncomfortable. I lie there, knowing I'm cocooned but somehow feeling immersed, with just the constant tap, tap, tapping in the chamber for company. I feel the tap as much as hear it, a tap-timbre in my head. I'm unsure if I'm hearing my own pulse beating to the rhythm of the scanner or whether the scanner's picking up my own resonance. It doesn't hurt or bother me, but it does exhaust me, so once more I drift away.

#

Back on the ward, other shifts of purposeful ants swarm my bed, only this time they're not harvesting from my body, but delivering. Whilst I sleep, they decorate my bedside with statuesque hardware – the straight regal staves and menacing hooks of IV infusion poles. Despite a hand which is already sore from the "let's try here" or "we'll just take a little more ...." cannula, a plastic, tubular body piercing fashionable in the realm of the seriously ill, the doctor wants to start antibiotics, so he's going straight for the jugular, as it were. He assures my children that this is standard treatment, despite the lack of diagnosis. So the nurses hook me up, hanging bags of crystal clear fluids – antibiotics with a saline chaser. It's shaping up to be something of a party, if only I could join in.

#

Others come, of course. The Visitors. Something of a family gathering occurs without me, but around me. In the recesses of my exhausted, infected brain, I think that I am dead, or at least dying. Whether I recognise them or not, these are my family, my siblings and my friends. They are gathered at my bedside. This can only mean one thing, can't it?

The wake
They come and come
Am I dying am I dead?
Like a wake
They talk with each other
Then a word to me
The flowers and cards
All gone now
And the people too

When actually more wakeful, I do try to join in, yet even in my moments of presence, the essential "me" remains absent. Instead, it seems that I am developing alternative ways of making some kind of presence felt, with personality traits which I've never had before. I've always been an agreeable and completely professional woman. Ok, so at the moment I don't exactly look like one, with my hospital gown and my new-found antipathy towards personal grooming, but my capacity is still that of my own pleasant, diplomatic person. Isn't it?

A lady arrives, someone I know well, apparently. She sits at my bedside patting my hand, the stereotypical hospital visitor you'd see in a sit-com: chattering away cheerfully, congenial to a fault and so irrepressibly bright she's almost aglow. I turn to my daughter.

"Wouldn't she get on your nerves?" I share, with something of a stage whisper.

The nurses don't escape this aspect of my changeling personality. I punctuate visiting hours by pointing out, at volume apparently, which of the nurses smell. I am told to keep my voice down and I acquiesce, at least for a while. But in truth, I don't really understand why. After all, I'm up close and personal with these people, or at least they are up close and personal to me, with their cold, hands-on care, their pricking, sticking and strapping of my body, so I catch their whiffs. I may not be able to think with clarity, understand with wisdom or even reason with rationality - and I certainly don't seem to be able to stop random thoughts from escaping my lips - but I can still pick up the aroma from the effects of a cheap deodorant in a polyester tunic. I experience it then I share it with any lucky listener who's around before it's then gone from my mind. This is evidently the modus operandi of the thief's victim, the new "me". Unfortunately though, what I share and then instantly forget appears to stick in the minds of others.

I don't just forget my own fair or foul words; I also forget what others have said to me. Evidently, like a goldfish in a bowl, I even forget who's been to see me - whether I recognise them or not. Visitor after well-meaning visitor repeats to me "of course you remember ... of course we had conversations, you were part of them!" When my pounding head allows, I ponder their absolute certainty of this from my bed. This "of course you remember" phrase of theirs becomes a familiar chant, as automatic a part of our conversations as "hello" and "goodbye". Someone other than me always knows better; I just don't seem to know or understand enough and I sure as hell don't remember.

At some point, a little boy appears in the bed opposite me. He does not seem ill to me, but then, I don't suppose I seem ill to him: I'm just an old, tired stranger in the bed opposite. He doesn't know that I'm not myself or that I'm actually a stranger to myself too. This, and the enforced companionship of the medical ward for the as-yet-undiagnosed, puts us on a level playing field for the game of trying to get better that seems to be going on around us.

He also doesn't know that I don't like fizzy drinks. I don't know that either, so when he offers to share, I gratefully accept both the bubbling rush of sugar and the gesture of friendship which, because I don't recognise my actual friends, seems both welcome and genuine: whilst my intellectual connection to my old friends has come adrift, I am secure in my infantile connection with my new friend.

That handsome, careworn looking man, who I'm told is my son, arrives to find me sipping Coca-Cola and colluding with an eight year old, probably about the smelly nurses. The scene might have seemed quite a positive one, except for the fact that apparently one of us is acting like a badly behaved child.

#

Whilst the faces in the beds opposite change around with disquieting frequency, the ward routine remains constant, punctuated by visits and tests. One of these is punctuation in a very literal way - a Lumbar Puncture. On the day of this test I'm tired and anxious: this illness and lack of progress with any aspect of diagnosis, treatment or recovery is exhausting me.

Despite my own crankiness, the two doctors are extremely pleasant to me and, although I don't retain much from day to day, I recall one of them from the previous day's round of testing. It's not his facial features which spark the tiny flicker of recall, but his colourful shirts. Of course, no sooner than the random recollection pops into my head, it also bursts forth from my lips. "No orange shirt today then?"

He's affable about this. "No, we have a different one for each day" he responds brightly. He smiles at me benignly whilst my son, who's travelled all the way from Ireland to visit me, looks lost and extremely hurt. I can see from his face, he finds it upsetting that I should be aware of a stranger's shirt when I've persistently failed to recognise him. His pain is caught somewhere in the space between us and I struggle to find the right words to comfort my own child. I try to think of some, but I'm so tired that even finding those wrong words, which I seem to have become quite good at when awake, is beyond me. I can only sleep my way through the test.

#

My children continue to pace, then sit and watch me sleep. I know I'm having a hard time of it, what with this feeling of complete displacement and confusion, as the rigours of this unknown condition ravage my body, but it's also hard for them. I'm aware that, like my new little friend in the bed opposite, you need your parents when you're in hospital – what you don't want is to have a parent *in* hospital. My children only have me and I'm the one in the bed whilst they hold my hand – it can't be me holding their hands. I'm not sure whether it's despite or because of my illness and confusion, but I'm aware that something's not right about this. My hospitalised hand is being held by the wrong ones ... I want my parents to come and look after me, don't they know I'm in the hospital?

Some vague stirring ignites - instinct or memory, I'm not really sure which, but it tells me that I am an orphan. This is not uncommon for someone of 57, I guess, but my 57 year old self is not the one in this bed, the thief has removed her and left this orphaned changeling in her stead. The orphan thought terrifies and confuses me – I don't know if what's happening is fact or illusion, or what form my release from this condition might take: I don't want my children to experience being orphans, yet I can't be a mother like *this*. I hold onto this terrifying thought as long as I can, until I'm able to spill it, in its swollen, tear-stained horror, all over the next consultant who wakes me: this stasis, this not getting better is not an option for me. Diagnose me, treat me, mend me – whatever it takes, return me to my children, to myself - or let me exit now.

Thankfully, it's the first part of this trio of progress which is achieved. After more inconclusive results, results which eliminate and results which concur or are tantalisingly "indicative", a diagnosis of Viral Encephalitis is agreed.

3. Trick or Treatment

The ceilings are moving once again. This time I'm off my trolley (with no small sense of irony) and travelling in my bed, en-route to a whole new ward which comes courtesy of at last having a diagnosis.

Of course, a ward's a ward: they all smell the same, look the same. They offer all the bland appeal of a budget hotel chain and have just as much emphasis on client comfort and hospitality. So it follows that in the true tradition of size of the chain being relative to level of care, I become lost in this bigger, noisier ward. I know I've just said that wards are all the same, but this new ward is a source of innumerable fears, both unknown: new patients, new consultant, new staff, new treatment; and those which are now despairingly familiar: carelessly inserted cannulas, bruised, painful hands and the infernal routines, of which ten doses of the intravenous anti-viral treatment form a significant part.

Part of me is glad to be here though, because it means progress. Having been asleep or "absent" through much of the diagnostic period, I'm now more wakeful. That is, my eyes, when closed, bring colour and thought, instead of complete oblivion. They are easier to open and, what's more, to keep open. Similarly my head, recently a throbbing life-force which seemed somewhat detached from the rest of me, feels closer to base. My limbs still have the approximate functional capacity of lead-lined spaghetti - elastically cooked or with the brittleness of the raw thing; either way works or not, as it happens. Still, they serve me, if not well then at least painfully and slowly.

I miss my juvenile companion of the previous ward and, when I'm having a less than confused moment, I realise that whilst my body holds the sense of being catapulted into senility, this itself is purely the physical experience of my illness. By contrast, my emotional reality is that I appear to have reverted to a very infantile stage. I find it hard to remember that I am a grown up. A parent. This latter understanding is of course made far more elusive by the fact I still cannot recognise my own dear son.

#

Along with the treatment, come the tricks which remind me I'm still a physical human being with obligations, such as attending to my grooming. Hospital showers are at best purely perfunctory. At worst they are degrading in a way that my Peter-Pan brain completely caves in over trying to understand. This context is created in no small part by my bizarre infantile emotional state and the apparent role-reversal with my daughter.

"Have you had a shower?"

"No" I reply, honesty being both the best policy and something which I appear not to be able to refrain from.

"You'd better then" I am told. With this, I am marched to the wet room. Sometimes, a little time is taken to disconnect me from my drip, whilst at other times it trails, still hanging from its hat stand-like contraption, me clutching it like a grasping, jealous companion or it holding me up and propelling me forwards, its squeaking wheels the only impetus for my undecided legs.

Showers continue to upset me. OK, so they're useful in a hurry, for that quick splash and dash, but I am a bath person ... correction, I am a lady of the bath. I enjoy my oils, the sensory caress of the fragrance, the hydration element to the skin, the soaking away of a day's physical and emotional ills, my me-time-bath-time. This aspect of my personality, enhanced by the muscle-memory and a bodily as well as instinctive aching for a long soak in the tub, has evidently not yet surrendered to the Encephalitis. However, the survival of a fully-intact preference is short-lived as it's relinquished in favour of the only resources available: it's shower or stink, and I am not permitted to stink.

I stand under the gush in a shivering huddle, despite the semi-warmth of the flow. I fear the water on my face. I don't know if this is a long-held terror from childhood or a new-found fear courtesy of my infantile encephalitic emotions. All I do know is that I dread the sensation of the deluge on my face, the unbearable stinging splash. This very real panic, coupled with the embarrassment of showering in front of my daughter does nothing to alleviate my fear of drowning – literally or metaphorically, within my current situation. This routine of relentless mortification continues to exhaust me and after each episode I drag myself, heaving my personal hat-stand complete with its not yet restorative handbag of fluids, back to my bed, perchance to sleep.

#

These are the early days, when I get away lightly with my grooming routine. At some point, I am given a deodorant to incorporate into the proceedings. Fuzzy from sleep and vague from viral overload, I hold it in my hands, unable for the life of me to figure out what to do with it. But apparently I am supposed to know. So, like a lab monkey given a human object to explore, I have no option but to try. The cap turns, muscle memory kicks in and I unscrew it successfully. Once it's open, I feel a sense of recognition, of understanding. I close my eyes and inhale. Creamy, fragrant, vaguely musky, like wet flowers. I have decided - it smells like hand-cream. Feeling inordinately pleased with myself, but not wanting to show quite how difficult this whole process has been, I proceed to use my hand-cream with purposeful nonchalance. Like the clumsy child I've become, I roll it onto the palms of my hands, until I am admonished in a tone of horror mixed with complete astonishment. Thus I re-learn all about roll-on deodorants; I'm shown exactly where and how I should be rolling it.

Yet I learn far more from this episode. One woman's deodorant, to mask her less-than-social bodily effects, is this woman's symbol of degeneration; re-learning to use it serves only to mask the strong stench of my decline. Now, I know exactly where I am and the thought terrifies me. I have been asleep in an academically "healthy" state for several weeks, yet now have to be shown how to use a deodorant. This incident becomes another mantra, another item on the "of course you remember ..." list. The thing is, I'm like a child who's never been shown: I don't remember at all.

Ignorance is reputed to be bliss of course and it would be delightful to be completely ignorant of my own shortcomings; there's little stress in being none the wiser. However, the IV fulfils its promise and, as my days and routines become extended by my periods of wakefulness, my short-comings become apparent. To say this is a worry is something of an understatement as, despite my lack of memory of basic processes, actions and everyday tasks, I cannot be ignorant of the fact that I am falling short of expectations – my own and others'.

I watch both the fretful, kind man who is my son and my tired, anxious daughter as, in turn, they watch me whilst pretending not to. Even with treatment underway, my illness continues to be so hard for them. We're in another situation where, quite rightly as my children, they expect better of me and I, quite wrongly in the reality of my condition, expect better of myself.

At times, my limitations are pointed out to me. Sometimes this is meant as an act of kindness, to remind me of a step missed out but more often my inabilities are highlighted with a sense of incredulity. It's incredible to me too. I don't have that cloak of ignorance to hide behind – instinct tells me that I'm supposed to know these basic routines yet, like a kid who hasn't revised for those big, completely unavoidable exams, I repeatedly fail. Still in the grip of my latest speak-first-moderate-your-thoughts-afterwards changeling persona, I find I cannot bear to have my inabilities discussed within my own earshot and I am forthright about this. Is a little restraint, or even discretion about it, too much to ask? I have enough to cope with in acknowledging all my inabilities to myself, pointing it out to me is, ironically, pretty pointless. Moreover, it's painful.

#

In this ward, I am now under the care of a different consultant. He's a lovely, professional man who always seems to be in a good mood. And that's not just by comparison to his overworked colleagues and the anxious, sick people around him; this man looks genuinely happy and his manner is calm, comforting and courteous. I'm secretly pleased with myself as I find I can remember his name easily. This might be seen as good progress but it's more to do with the fact that his name's the same as a famous brand of vacuum cleaner. Strangely, and certainly unforgivably in the context of my own poor son, this brand and thus the doctor's name, seems to remain with me. As such, despite the scramble in my head and my inability to recall who my own child is, I remember this doctor faultlessly. So, when he greets me by name, I can reciprocate like my old professional self, as if we were meeting ... well, for a meeting. I'm very pleased about this, although I don't reveal my method to him; I guess I'm not the first to remember him for his dust-busting name-sake.

Besides, I'm sure he's not interested in my recall of his name – he has other questions on his seemingly ceaseless list: Prime Minister's name? Queen's name? Year? Month? Day? Date? My efforts are exhausting, but I am pleased with my responses – I recall a lot ... the Queen is Victoria, this I know for fact. Questions are followed by physical interrogation: push hands, up, down, out, away, in.... I'm good at this too I'm sure, this medical hokey-kokey. Despite my linguine limbs I push up and away as instructed – at least as much as the IV paraphernalia and my limited wakefulness permits.

#

Wakefulness and sleep have become another issue altogether on this ward. Despite the lookie-likie sameness of these wards, this new ward has subtle differences which come with its size and arrangement. I notice it during the day, from the sensory overload which comes with its intrusive sterile light and the acoustically amplified clamour and clatter from the combined industries of care and cleanliness. Yet despite this auditory excess, which makes my head throb and my ears sing, ring and whistle, I welcome the daytime on this ward: the night-time, the dark, is another matter entirely.

The hospital routine is now well embedded, along with its expectations; when the ward settles to sleep, so should I. Yet what I experience is not sleep, it's not restful. I find myself trapped in a place which falls between sleeping and waking, where dreams are reality and reality is a brutal, hallucinogenic harbour for the fears which have come to berth on the Encephalitic tide. In its relentless pillage of my persona, the thief has left the drawers and doors of all the hidden areas of my brain carelessly, clumsily open, allowing the disturbing thoughts and childhood fears, once well locked away, to run loose in my brain.

By day and in wakefulness my brain is of course kept very busy. It's full of my new learning of the expected behaviours and routines of basic grooming and communication, the re-establishment of this new form of my 'self', whoever I am. This busy-ness of my daytime brain in trying to repair the devastation to my physical condition is what could be deemed "Another Good Thing" that is, it protects me from the worst of the destruction of my emotional being.

But at night, during those hours of darkness when I should be resting and letting the cure run its course as it's pushed from plastic pouch to white cells, racing, rejuvenating and partying through my veins, the remaining contents of my ravaged brain run amok like a hoodlum with a spray can and a poor attitude, who's just one step ahead of the cells in white armour. Each night, as the main lights of the ward are switched off, the shadowed corners of the room encroach and the pillars which support the ceiling by day serve only as hiding places for the monsters in the blackness beyond. From these blurred shadows come rats, bats, ghouls and ghosts of monochrome, or mainly white. The dim lighting of the nurses' station and the supposedly comforting glow of the subdued safety lights illuminate my tormentors in negative relief, rendering them not only more visible but also far more gruesome.

#

It's the night of February 8th and my day has, like all of them, been one long round of trying to get better in two distinct senses: better enough and not worse. One by one, the lights go out for bedtime, for rest time. Instantly my enemies gather. I have a sense, a very strong sense, of being in a horsebox. The air is thick with vermin, both those that I can see and those that I can feel, their eyes upon me. Nothing is said – despite the many childish reversions I do have, these nightmare creatures aren't included. These are no Scooby Doo baddies, none of the wailing and gnashing of childhood ghosties, no obvious menace of the stealthy, child-shrieking "I'm coming to get you" kind.

What there is instead is a palpable intent to instil fear. It permeates me as easily as the intravenous infusion. It's within my strangled throat and heaving chest – it is here, it is real and it has me trapped. The confines of my bed, the tangled knots of sheets add to this sense of entrapment. I see the spectres all around the pillars as they encroach. They are white, elongated sea shells with pointed, protruding faces and long loose tentacles flowing behind them. Their presence makes no sense and renders me insensible in equal measures.

In my head and with my eyes, I try to move away, to see beyond them but although they don't follow, the somewhere else my mind takes me to is just as confusing, just as scary. I'm in Wimbledon, in a shop opposite the railway station. Yet that can't be, because I find myself exiting the shop onto a street I know well, a street in Sutton. I go back and forth – Sutton, Wimbledon. Over on the Wimbledon side I am given a tonic. It's a glass of very yellow juice for an infection or something. Only it is the colour of pustular infection itself. I don't want it. I mustn't have it. I scan the room for assistance, but see only rows of tables with lots of people waiting for this treatment, waiting to access that endless little cubicle with its glasses of bile toned tonic, the colour of illness.

This sense of coming and going around me continues, just like the bustle of London, the heave of the masses on a mission, the rush-hour surge. Carried in their wake, a true state of wakefulness, I find myself in Putney and I know that the crowds who tug me in their tow are taking me to the sanatorium. Even as I am stricken with a fear which is absolute in its relentlessness, something is colliding. There's a battle between the physical fear which constricts my throat and limbs and the vaguest sense of rationality which tells me that there are nurses here to help. They are over there, at the nurses' station. Despite the gauntlet of ghouls and vermin around me (I feel them behind and above my bed, waiting for their chance), I resolve to get help from the nurses before the worst happens and I am dragged off in the surge to the sanatorium.

I have to launch myself, from the relative safety of my bed and into the shadows of my horrors: the curtained passages between the beds, the pillars, the sleeping humps in the other beds – the other patients' oblivion protecting them from the evils which are roaming the ward, hiding behind their very beds. I shuffle carefully, purposefully to the nurses' station and manage to tell the nurse that I need to talk to my daughter.

"It's very late, she'll be in bed," the nurse tells me, turning her attention back to the computer, oblivious to the laughing wisps of evil over her shoulder, the rats on the counter.

"She told you that you could ring if I needed her." This is an important snippet of a conversation carried out around me, about me. I've managed to retain it and I don't hesitate to use it. Tears, as much as fear, are now starting to replace the blood in my body. I'm running high, I'm running scared, I wish to God that I could run in reality.

I turn to the next nurse to appeal for help, but am taken aback, horrified. As she turns to acknowledge me, I realise that something's not right with her, or perhaps it is even less right with me. This nurse has one normal and one very small arm. In her white tunic, with her long arm and short arm she completes my fear: the phantoms can do everything; they have taken over not only the darkness of the ward, but also the light.

"What ... what happened to your arm?" I don't know if I'm trying to catch the creature out in its trick, or whether my uninhibited verbosity now extends to gossiping with ghouls, engaging with the entities which are taking over the normality of the ward. What is she, with her white robes and her non-matching arms?

The nurse tells me, very quietly and calmly, that she was born this way. I can't stop myself. For this to be her "reality" amongst the surreal circus going on about us is too much. I ask her how she manages and she, still courteous despite the smirking shell-shapes floating up, around and behind her, explains. I admire her calmness, her fortitude. It is catching. I start to feel calmer too, until I realise that the first nurse has made no effort to reach for the phone, to contact my daughter.

My fear explodes. In a tangle of tears I scream at her to make the call, just make the call, it's all I want. "She's my daughter, she said call her, she'll understand!" I scream until hysteria gives way to hoarseness, until the phone is picked up, the number dialled and the message imparted. I don't know where I am, where I end up in the meantime. I know I don't return to my bed with its terrors scrambling around the curtains and I don't think I stay at the nurses' station, the scene of my most complete loss of dignity so far. I'm nowhere until my daughter arrives.

My relief upon seeing her is total. Physically and emotionally I surrender to her protection, the weight of fear upon me diminished merely by her presence. She takes me to the day room where we lay on the sofa, waiting for the ghosts to creep off or the dawn to creep in, either is enough for me. Sam comforts me, mothers me, as she soothes the savage, swollen ugliness of pure and very real fear from my face. Meanwhile my nocturnal stalkers, content with their moment of triumph, disperse. Physically I gain confidence and strength from Sam's presence, yet I stay frightened. Even in my worse dreams, my childhood nightmares of scary monsters, I've never experienced anything so real, so frightening. Perhaps it's because I've been so clearly awake whilst it's all been happening around me or maybe it's because I've found that surreality is actually a real place that can entrap you with its web of lies and deceit, I just don't know. Yet I do know that whilst nothing touched me, everything chilled my core. My very soul is scared.

When I am calmer, when the ghouls, the rats and the bats have retreated to wherever it was they came from (please God don't let it have been from within me), I tell Sam to go home to her family, to get some rest. I guess we'll discuss it later, but right now, we both need some proper sleep. So I am tucked back up in bed, a childhood prayer away from the oblivion I now crave ... now as I lay me down to sleep, I pray the Lord my soul to keep and should I die, before I wake ... that's really OK by me. I've had enough, I can't do this anymore.

4. Carefully Does It

I'm still here - physically, I mean, as opposed to metaphysically in response to my daily prayer to be allowed to just stop playing this game. And of course I mean literally still *here*, in the hospital, where I can't keep track of the passing days despite the fact they are punctuated abruptly by those endless, infested nights.

Likewise, just as I continue to fear my nights, I also still lack the words to explain in any way that others can really understand, much less sympathise with, what happens as darkness falls. Instinct tells me there's a lack of understanding on my part too ... I can't really understand why everyone else can't see what I see, but then I realise it's because I haven't asked them. The same instinct which reminds me of my own lack of understanding seems to be trying to protect me ... I don't want them to think I'm mad, so I'm keeping my insights and sightings to myself, in the hope that someone else will mention it. But they don't.

#

February continues and a routine (of sorts) has developed ... around me, for me and possibly with me, although I don't recall the conversations that I apparently had, the actions I supposedly agreed to.

"Of course you remember!" remains the team mantra, from those staff and family who I see from day to day. I suspect everyone of some complicity and it's exhausting, this trying not to be caught out, keeping tabs on what's being done, being said.

I know they think I'm being awkward and neither they (nor I for that matter) understand quite why it should be so. Seriously, is it being awkward to want to know what's going on? To want to know what's being said and planned? Beneath my veil of apparent awkwardness, thin as this hospital bed sheet, lies my fear; I don't know what happened to me in these past weeks and I don't know what's happening to me now. For sure, there are conversations, many conversations apparently, when I'm told what's going on, but no sooner are they spoken than the words and their meaning have floated away, so I have to ask and then keep asking, which appears to be awkward for everyone.

#

It's lunchtime, or rather what I really mean is it's time for the lunchtime lurch of the stomach. Although the sound of a trundling trolley could herald the arrival of one of many hundreds of possible hospital trolleys with different purposes, I know instantly that it's the food one by the smell. Yes, it's one of those, I can smell it long before I see it and my stomach flips in anticipation, but not in a good way. No excitement here or even hunger for that matter, just dread.

Yes, it's safe to say that I don't like the hospital food. I stare at each platter as it's placed before me by a member of staff, complete with a cursory, no-eye-contact smile. I regard the messed up meals but can identify what I'm expected to eat only by colour. I don't know if this is the fault of the catering or my current word-finding ability, but I choose to blame the catering. The predominant colours are brown and green, although not warm browns, or fresh greens, but the paint palette hues of unidentifiable mixtures and mistakes. The only safely recognisable foods are the cheese and biscuits in their cheerful little packs. I feel safe with these and take them quickly, even if I don't feel like eating them. I stash them in my locker for later, when I might be hungry.

Because she knows how I feel about the catering, Sam brings me food - sometimes a meal or fresh sandwiches. It seems that I'm also awkward about this, but I don't really know how that happens. She brings me a sandwich, made with lovely seeded bread and it actually appeals to me, I feel hungry in my stomach and in my anticipating mouth. I eat it with gusto, thank her profusely and tell her I love the seedy bread. Later on, she brings me another and I tell her I need her to change it because I don't like that bread.

"I only bring it because you like it," she replies, clearly confused and exasperated.

"Well, I don't anymore." And truly I don't, now.

#

What else is there to break up the days? Visiting time, of course. My son's had to return to Ireland but in his stead, two of my sisters have come over. As they arrive to visit me I'm looking out of the window, at the view across the way of other ward windows and this seems to create a strange kind of background as they greet me. I am struck by their smart appearance, which makes them appear very business-like, unexpectedly so against the sterile backdrop of the ward and the blank stare of window upon window. I'm reminded that I too am a business woman, but I can't see it in myself. In fact, no-one would see it in me, at the moment. It scares me, the idea that anyone who already knows me, knows what I am (or should that be was?) is comparing what they now see to that person. Worse though, is the idea that anyone new, the doctors, other patients, their visitors, don't know any of that; they don't see that person, just this one, the one that isn't me, the one that's still "not herself."

I find visitors tiring, although I want them to come. I don't look forward to much here, apart from visitors coming in or getting out myself. At the moment, there's no sign of me going anywhere, so everyone comes to me and then goes again although I can't always remember who's been, or when. Everything merges like a cinematic montage which captures moments in time before fading to a new scene.

I recognise evening visiting though. As it's February, by the time evening visiting comes around, darkness is already looming outside. Often, the ghouls don't wait for the ward lights to dim, or my visitors to leave. Instead, the rats scurry around, whilst the ghouls skim across the curtains, floor and ceiling. Their strategy, devious in the extreme, is to lurk behind the unwitting visitors. They don't draw attention to themselves from anyone else but I see them, watching me. My visitors go, assuming they're leaving me in good spirits, not realising that I remain surrounded by evil ones. Like me, they're here for the night.

#

Another little break comes when the weather's reasonable and my legs amenable, because this means that I can, with the help of various aids and appliances, accompany Sam and Evie for a jaunt to the hospital lake. We take our lunch there, enjoying watching the simple life of the ducks, and the to and fro of the staff, busy people with busy lives, whilst my own is on hold.

#

The days continue. Never my favourite month, this February seems eternal. The daily routine of pricking, testing and scanning continues, although in truth there are elements I don't mind about this. Trips on trolleys or in wheelchairs to other departments for scans and MRIs are little outings, welcome breaks from the confines of the ward. I am transported, just for a short time and have the chance for contact with somebody new even if just for a few minutes. Although the exhaustion and headaches continue, I do my best to make the most of these excursions.

One of the more annoying pains I can't avoid though, is from my hand, where the cannula lurks. Although welcome, as the portal for the drugs which should help me to get better, the site itself is painful mess, my hand mock-monochrome hues of black, blue and various shades of yellow. I watch carefully to see which trolley the staff approach me with, to know whether to steel myself for the onslaught of pricking and stabbing.

One of the junior doctors is coming, armed with both her instruments of torture and a wan smile of empathy.

"I hate to do this to your poor hand, it looks so sore," she says.

But despite her admission, she carries on with the task, literally in hand. Although she's awful at it, she's not the worst. Now I'm not a feeble woman, I've given birth, I've struggled with this explosive head, but I cry when the phlebotomists swoop like vampires for their blood fix, leaving my arm curiously both pale yet colourful from their painful attention.

One of the Filipino nurses is best at replacing the cannulas. When she's on shift in the mornings I try to catch her eye, before the doctors come around, hoping that if I'm lucky she'll be able to come over and pop a fresh one in before they arrive. Reassuringly kind and amazingly deft, she pops the needle in place within a split second, unlike others who take ages with their prodding and poking as they try, in vain for a place in vein, scraping the inside of my hand with the spiteful needle, causing bruises like tattoos across the back of my hand.

#

I'm trying not to be passive in my recovery. My new event, both to break the monotony and to prove myself improved, is to take regular shuffles to the day room. Although my stance is duck-like and my gait painfully slow and unbalanced, this room, at the end of the corridor, becomes a personal challenge as it seems to embody my own contrasts and conflict:

* I like being here because it's something I can do, a choice I can make independently. Yet, I don't like the room. It seems to reflect everything I am at the moment: drab but trying to be functional, albeit in some outdated, forgotten form.

* I like that when I'm here I can pretend to myself that all's normal by trying activities such as making myself a drink, yet I dislike that to do so I have to watch myself as if I'm outside of my body. I see my hands try to pick up a cup or replace the tea pot, clumsy as a clown. I'm slow and shaky, every movement an exaggerated effort, a slow-motion, frame-by-frame version of usual, everyday activities. It's inexplicable, but noticeable. I think I should ask the doctors about this, but I know that I won't remember to do so, by the time I've baby-stepped back to my bed.

* I like that I can use the room to see "baby girl". We sit on the sofa and play, which seems to be what normal grandmothers would do. She smiles, gurgles and laughs at me, so I laugh too. Yet I dislike that when she goes, I cry. I cry the fat, snotty tears of the forgotten; I'm so troubled by my loss, of my limited knowledge of her and of what she will know of me, this person that I seem to be.

#

The days are passing slowly and I'm trying to think of more things I might do, both to pass the time and to show that I can achieve things, that I can manage. I ask Sam to bring some nail varnish in so that I can complete elements of my personal care for myself. Most of the time I'm confused and lethargic, but I'm not about this; I have a strong sense of wanting to normalise the awful hospital-enforced necessities, such as the desperate, on-going indignity of my showering routine. I'm missing a routine of getting dressed for work, for social events and for myself. The arrival of the nail varnish helps, both to lift my spirits and to pass the time.

Or at least that's the theory. The practice of course is rather different. When the nail varnish arrives, I know that I've got neither the ability nor the energy to do anything with it. It sits on the cabinet as a reminder of my passing thought, the whimsy of the woman I used to be. After a few days of its silent, shiny taunting, I decide to give it a go. This is a bad move. My first attempts are like a child's finger painting, literally. These attempts have to be removed immediately, by the same shaking hands which created the mess, until I can get someone to help me.

The junior doctors seem to find this fun. One of them jokes with me about being the lady whose nails match her pyjamas. I don't know why this pleases me so, but it does. It's good to be "seen" – I'd rather match my pyjamas than just blend into these sterile, blank walls which seem to reflect my own weary nothingness.

#

The same lovely house doctor comes each day with his entourage; he always greets me with "good morning, Mrs Scott" which makes such a difference. I don't know which of me he sees, this sick one or a glimpse of the woman I used to be, but the fact he addresses me at all as a person means everything to me. His charm is infectious and means I have something to look forward to, a tiny break from the monotony of the ward, plus there's always the chance that he'll have something positive or useful to share.

At some point, a neurologist joins the rounds. Actually, I think he's been part of the entourage for a while but as an unobtrusive, observing presence. Now he too seeks to establish a form of human contact – that is to say, he actually makes eye contact as he talks to me. He offers smiles and nods sagely so that I know I'm not talking gibberish when they ask me their questions. And they do still ask a lot of questions. I never know why, but I do my best to answer before they're off again, on their way.

#

It's on the back of one of these visits that I decide that lists and notes might help, to resolve the confusion in my mind and what seems to be something of a creeping inability to fully hear, let alone remember what everyone is saying to me. Sam brings me a pen and a pad and I settle on the bed, with that standard hospital bed-table organised in front of me, ready to write my first list.

Like my activities in the day room, the effort is immense. Those motor-controlled split-second instructions from brain to fingers seem to miss their beat. The pen's on the paper but the words I've trapped in my head, ready to write down, won't appear on the page. Instead, I regard the ill-formed scribbles of a toddler let loose with a crayon. Confusion and fear rise again. Am I not writing properly, therefore can't read it properly or am I out of practice with my reading too and my writing's not too bad? There seems to be only one way to find out without having to ask someone else, someone who might judge my scribbles as a reflection of myself.

So, on my next shuffle to the dayroom, I pick up a magazine and flick through it eagerly, waiting to be absorbed and reassured by the delights within. Yet there's no familiarity within its pages, just photographs of "famous" people I don't recognise. In comparison to my own inept scrawl, the magazine holds fully formed, clear print letters, beautifully constructed to convey whole words, meanings and communications. Yet I can't decipher them with any kind of familiarity or recognition. Each one jigs and jumbles, almost playing charades as it tries to convey its meaning, share its joy. The odd word that I can decipher then dances away before I can recall what it's saying, fully understand its denotation. And as for connotation? Tears plop silently onto the page. I have no memory base for my own child, let alone others' words. I'm alone in a meaningless world.

#

Later, back on the ward, I have another idea. I'll ask Sam to bring me my laptop. She brings it on her next visit so, once again with the bed-table serving as my desk, I settle into the opportunity to reassure myself that a little practice and focus is all I'll need. I pin down some of the words floating in my head and painstakingly locate the keys for each letter. I'd like to think that I'm tickling the keys in my usual professional manner, but I can see for myself the slow motion of my finger to key action. There's no gentle, productive tapping, but a resolute and painfully slow process of identifying the letter I need in my head, then trying to match it on the keyboard and press it before the thought slips away. Alternatively, when I can't think of the letter I need, I peer at the keyboard for inspiration, trying to absorb each letter's role and purpose in life and match it to the word I'm thinking of. I use the ones which seem to fit, jabbing at the keyboard like a drunkard wearing boxing gloves. Sam and I look at what I have written, but it isn't what I wrote, it's the drunkard's words instead. I can't take my eyes off the page, at that semantically meaningless but personally significant stream-of-barely-consciousness. I'm still not myself ... I'm an inadequate, frustrated version of me and, what's more, I am truly disgusted with this new person. I feel bile rise in my chest, just as tears seem to gather somewhere at the back of my throat. I banish the page from my sight, or rather, make Sam delete it.

#

I find myself in my bed, crying. Sometimes I know it's happening: I feel sad, my face tingles with the effort of suppression and, as my usual lethargy gains the upper hand, the effort ceases and the tears flow. At other times, I don't feel anything, just so very tired. I try to nap, yet tears creep upon me sooner than sleep, but bringing no comfort, just release and moment of hiatus where I don't have to try to be anything, least of all "myself."

The nurses offer no comfort either. Their busy-ness in all manner of practical, medical matters seems to render them oblivious to the silent, emotional responses of their patients. Any loud, angry explosions of emotion from the occasional, more aggressive patient are quickly dealt with, usually through those practical and definitely pharmaceutical means, but those others of us feeling all at sea: emotional, tired and confused? We lie in our beds, waves of tears washing through the ward and no life boat between us.

I pray to go home and, much as a complete recovery and my own four walls would suit, I know it's not the comforts of my physical home that I'm really praying for. What I really crave now is to be taken to my eternal home. To die holds a distinct appeal as most of the time it seems to be far and away the easiest option. I'm so tired. I think I could easily just float away and cease to exist, after all, the life that was mine is no longer mine, the life I once owned has deserted me, along with my writing, reading and memory and it's exhausting this effort, this trying to keep doing things the hard way, but I can't seem to stop myself. Someway, somehow, I have to keep trying.

#

At some point, nuns appear at the foot of my bed. Whilst I don't trust my eyes or my ears … or many of my faculties and senses, come to that, I trust the fact that because my children are standing and talking to the nuns, I can be sure the figures in grey and greyer are real. They certainly seem to be, as they turn to me with their kindly faces to introduce themselves. When they ask me my name I am inordinately pleased to think that, like the consultant, they care about me, about what's happening to me. I watch as they prepare a communion and share their sympathies with my children yet as the conversation progresses, I'm aware that although I'm the main attraction at this event, *I* am superfluous … I have become "she" and "her". Something is starting to grate within me as, although I'm confused about many things, one thing becomes clear to me – they have forgotten my name.

Despite the fact that these ladies embody faith, love and forgiveness, I'm finding their error unforgivable. I don't know where it's coming from, this rising anger but I know where it's going: instinctively I want to snarl and recoil from the nuns' benevolence, their healing thoughts and prayers.

My children can't understand my behaviour, my reactions. Does it really matter? Indeed, does it *really* matter? Well that's like asking if *I* really matter – the whole thing matters to me! When they ask my name, I take this as interest, as genuine concern, yet in reality it's just a passing courtesy, not even a sincere one, to another nobody in a bed, another name on their list amongst many more. Of course it's unreasonable to expect them to remember every person, match every name to a face on their once-a-week pastoral visit. Yes, I realise it probably is unreasonable, but unreasonable appears to be something I *can* do.

#

Many days pass this way: tiredness and tears; trial and error to find out what I can do; identify what seems to have slipped away. With reading and writing off the entertainment schedule, I'm left with just visitors, the other patients and the TV or radio, as well as some well-deserved naps, to break the monotony of these days. Apart from the naps though, all those other options are giving rise to another discovery.

The TV seems pretty nonsensical at the best of times, to be honest, but as well as not being able to fully understand or remember what's said, I find I can't really seem to hear it very well. There's plenty of noise alright, like I'm listening to a wind storm, but discernable words are difficult to keep track of; when others speak or I try to listen to the TV, the words and sounds have to compete with the storm in my ears.

This seems to affect everything and of course, when I'm talking to the doctors it's the same, so at least I do remember to mention it. I mention it to all of them, the consultants, the affable junior doctor, nurses and eventually one of the days is broken up with a new outing, to the audiologists for a hearing test. I am given a piece of paper with the results, which someone tries to explain to me:

"The audiogram showed bilateral sensori-neural hearing loss for all frequencies down 40 to 50 dB."

These results add to the growing sense of numbness, of invisibility which seems to shroud me. No one seems to have anything to say about whether this is permanent or not and I don't really know who to ask, as it seems the results have absolved this hospital of any further action with regards to my hearing. Instead, I am given a letter of referral to St George's in Tooting for further assessment, with the instruction that I am to get in touch with them after discharge. The twist of this double-edged blade eases somewhat as I realise I now have something of a landmark on the bleak landscape of my calendar: discharge.

The word continues to pop up in conversations with me, about me and apparently within those "of course you remember" conversations. At some point, I seem to recognise that maybe I just don't hear some of the things that are said to me, but I forget to share this. Still, maybe someone else will think of it, will realise? They don't.

I pick up on the words “care” and “supervision” as these seem to be involved in the latest planning. I interrogate them in my aching head, trying to uncover what these words and those colluding over them are saying about me. With a clarity which almost makes me laugh, I finally catch on to the fact that I’ll be allowed to go home so long as I stay with my daughter. We get on well enough, Sam and I, that’s not a problem, the main issue is my medical situation and pitiful, weak state. A compromise is reached: a trial weekend out with my daughter prior to my discharge.

The prospect seems like a dream, although I can see Sam, the doctors and nurses preparing and planning for it so I know that it’s real, it’s going to happen and I start to feel less lonely and more purposeful. The ward seems to take on a new shape and colour as a result; it’s bathed in the light of this new knowledge, this exciting prospect of release. I embrace this fluttering inside me as something close to happiness and it stays with me all the way to the hospital exit as I’m trundled along by a chirpy-chappy porter towards my first taste of freedom in well over a month.

5. In and Out

It's funny how things work out though. Over this weekend I've become horribly aware that I'm truly incapacitated, physically, emotionally and ... well, individually. Don't get me wrong, I was so excited about coming out and all that the weekend would hold, although even that started off in a weird, not-really-there kind of way. Even as the hospital prepared to discharge me for the weekend, the ever charming Welsh-lilting consultant gently joked with me about the major international rugby match between Ireland and Wales being at the heart of why I'm keen to be released.

"I don't know," he teased. "We're just letting you out so you can watch the rugby ...!"

What's rugby? I sit pondering this. What is it, and why would I want to watch it? In the event, two of my brothers and my nephew come over from Ireland to see me and of course the rugby does turn out to be a focal point for the afternoon. They sit, bookends on the couch whilst I sit on the armchair. So this is rugby. This is being at home. Yet of course I'm not at home, we're all of us in the warmth of my daughter's home, yet I can't seem to find my place in it.

OK, so I chose to sit over here in the armchair, but I have no choice really. Since the incontinence shows no sign of stopping, I'm self-conscious about odours, so feel obliged to remain slightly removed from others. And my hearing doesn't help. Conversation is arduous and exhausting and my anxiety over missing out or muddling up exacerbates it all. Instead of sharing the joy of this supposedly big event, the rugby match, the very game itself seems to epitomise my situation of just trying to keep up, hang on to the ball of sensibility before I'm tackled to the ground by exhaustion or a scrum of sensory interference makes me lose it completely. Alternatively, from my detached position of the armchair, I could be the winger, far outside and unable to keep up with the action. I'm the one who no-one wants to pass the ball to because I'll fumble, I'll flap, I just won't get it.

I feel sick to my stomach to realise what's happened; the thief has taken my joy. When there's humour, others laugh but I can't join in, I can't hear or understand. Most of all, I just don't find it funny.

It's become clear that my lack of joy isn't limited to expressions of humour and fun either. There's joy in appreciation; this I know from the woman I was before. I could appreciate and be appreciated in return, for kindnesses, for sharing, for wisdom, for the simple things in life and also those grand things which build finances, families and futures – I've always been one to acknowledge and appreciate. But when I'm in this armchair, an enforced appreciation is expected: I'm out of hospital, albeit for a weekend and for that I must be truly grateful. It's clear that I'm expected to appreciate this fact and for my face and my humour to show it: I'm out of hospital, hurrah! I must be on the mend, yippee! But I don't feel mended. I can't hear, can't laugh, can't realise that I need the toilet until it's regrettably too late. I can't appreciate being on the mend, when I still feel so very broken.

#

So it shouldn't surprise me when, at the end of the weekend, as I'm transferred back into my hospital bed, an extraordinary and inexplicable sense of relief grasps me in a warm hug. Yet the feeling pulls me up short, compromises me: I hate this ward, but I can't deny the sense of safety I feel about being here. Yes, it's still scary, it's still a lair full of rats and ghouls, but now I know that they follow me to Sam's house too, that they will find me wherever I am, some of my fear of the ward itself has given way to a sense of reprieve. Being plopped into a domestic setting, even for such a short time, has revealed many of my inabilities, hidden by the hospital's suspension of daily life as anyone knows it, with a sharp clarity. More than this though, I've found that expectation that I will rise to the occasion of being "better" far more frightening than many of the ghouls who presume to haunt me.

#

However, despite my own misgivings and the grim reality that although I am somewhat recovered (comparatively speaking, you understand) I am by no means "better", the weekend is deemed a success. On the face of it that's true – nothing calamitous happened, certainly not on my part and, as far as I know, for Sam and her family too. So, on the back of all this positivity, plans are made to discharge me into Sam's care where my hospital routine is to be played out on a different stage.

#

So here I am, I've been allowed home, but not to my own home. I'm tucked up, up and away in the spare upstairs bedroom because I'm literally, as well as personally, out of it most of the time. At first, this being mostly bed-ridden is fine to some extent because coming out of hospital with that ongoing expectation to be recovered is, for the most part, exhausting. But before long, with the expectation towards recovery and my own determination to build upon this at some level, I try to keep up with my daily shuffle. Unfortunately now my relentless drag to the day room has been exchanged for long, painful trips downstairs for meals. The stairway seems extraordinarily steep to me, not helped I suppose by the effect of my ears and hearing on my balance. The treads seem to move like an escalator, although without the helpful impetus of actually transporting me from up to down and back again. At the moment, I cannot tackle the stairs unaided, but have to wait for Sam or Simon or a visitor to help me. Their helpfulness is kind and purposeful "don't want you back in hospital, do we?" but makes me feel even more bereft of my own abilities, and sensibilities, in equal measure. These trips take so long, it seems I'm barely back in bed before it's time to go back down again.

Family meals take place pretty much in the same format as the rugby match. I'm a bystander at my own party, finding affinity only with the precious baby girl in her high chair. I cannot resist returning her uncomprehending smiles with my own - she's the only one who doesn't approach me with that "are you better yet?" expression, that need for things to be back to normal. I am normal to her, at least.

But I'm fooling no one else, least of all myself. Ok, I'm well aware that I should be, and indeed am, making an extreme effort to be, if not much better then at least on the mend, now that I'm out of hospital. But something's not right. I'm sitting here, at the dinner table, forcing smiles at the baby, forcing the fork towards my mouth whilst all the time the thought of eating is making my insides collapse. Not just the now-familiar incontinent sensation of fluids in free-fall, more that I have a liquid self and cannot take on solids at all.

I give up the meal early, with apologies … my poor daughter's trying so hard to make life normal and meals appetising, to build me up, but I have to return to my bed.

Of course, it's not that easy. First, the stairs present their arduous slog and, once their pinnacle is finally reached, there's a statutory trip to the bathroom. After all of the exertion, the down, then up again I have to, yet again, change my incontinence pads. There's a routine for this, but I can't remember what it is. I sit on the toilet as long as possible, head in my hands, waiting for my insides to quieten, my body to make a decision. At some point, I summon the strength to dispose of my old pad in the bin and fit a new one within my industrial-strength underwear. By the time I finally return to my room and gratefully sink into the waiting bed, I know two things: one is that my body has made its decision and the other? I know I won't be seeing downstairs again for a while.

I do, however, see start seeing the bottom of the bucket instead. It appears at regular intervals, intermittently at first and then constantly, as I roll helplessly under the duvet. Of course, I don't see the bottom of it for long, before it's covered with the dreary sludge and bitter splash of relentless sickness. This same-old scenario takes on the deja-vue of visitors who come and go as before, along with the rats and ghouls who gather every dusk to ensure that they still have me in their grip, whilst my own grasp is firmly on the necessary receptacles, the only things which stand between myself and a complete and utter decline of laying in a bed full of my own disgusting bodily emissions. I last for five days of vomiting, groaning and sobbing, before an ambulance comes to return me to yet another ward.

#

I'm only in the ward for one day, before they send me back to Sam's again, content that my state is "just" a minor pothole on that fine road to recovery which lies ahead of me. This flit from hospital to Sam's, Sam's to hospital does not lessen my confusion and what seems to be a growing anxiety.

It doesn't help my physical situation either. My body's distress signal doesn't lessen despite the "minor" significance attributed to it by the hospital. I can do nothing but recline and decline in Sam's spare bedroom. Once again, the thought strikes me that to close my eyes for one last time, against it all, may not be such a bad thing. And so, willingly, I close my eyes.

#

I open them to find myself back in the hospital once more, this time with no relief but a burning sense of absolute shame, a real sense of failure.

What's worse, is that this feeling of failure is not the only thing which is different. There's something else. It's not the aesthetics, the environment, despite the fact that I've now popped up in yet another ward, with a new bed and different companions, each with their varying complaints to adjust to, conversations to listen to (albeit in a muted tones) and of course to witness first-hand the worst indignities of their symptoms.

And it's not the routine, which persistently, almost defiantly, offers the same monotony, the same regime of tests and needles, of soreness, confusion and tiredness, with pauses only for more visitors or the arrival of platters of unidentifiable nutrition. I'm sick to my stomach, not just in that pervasive illness way or even in a literal vomiting way, just so sick of all of this.

That's the thing, that's what's different: I feel worse now, worse than I did before I was discharged. I'm sure I was more aware then, I felt like I was on the road to recovery albeit in a slow, relative way, but now? Now I've come off the road, I'm in a ditch somewhere, crashed and burned.

#

My senses continue to play havoc with me – I see things flitting around from the corners of my eyes, I can't hear properly as conversations are lost to the storms in my ears. And I smell something too, something warm and obnoxious. Convinced that all of my senses are in collusion to persuade me I'm going off my head, I mention it to one of the nurses who, to my surprise and (for the first time in a long time) delight, not only agrees with me but also explains it to me, "it's aviation fuel from the helipad." This new ward is downwind, it seems, from this vital emergency facility.

I play with this information, turning it over in my head, talking it over to myself and anyone else who will listen, "aviation fuel from the helipad." Despite the fact that the smell is proved to me not to be an illusion, its source takes on a mystical, metaphorical quality and the stench itself morphs from being obnoxious to holding a strange allure: aviation fuel from the helipad, the smell of outside, of journeys, of freedom, of life before.

The trouble is, I don't feel the same way about freedom any more. It occurs to me, one grey afternoon, that freedom has become one of those "be careful what you wish for" things. From this most recent experience of the road to recovery, boomeranging between the hospital and Sam's, I'm getting the awful feeling that being in hospital is probably the easy part – because trying to get better outside of it is certainly not an easy task. Once again my thoughts are side-tracked by the random roguish idea that, ironically, life would be easier if I could just die.

#

It's now March 2nd. I've been trying to walk more today, to re-establish a routine of shuffles to the dayroom. Although it's a different day room, its role and purpose are the same as far as I'm concerned. However, the difference in the scenario is *me*. Something's wrong with my walk. At some point, between being discharged and returned, my shuffle has become a waddle. I see my feet and watch incredulously as they move me along by shifting my body from one foot to the other, one foot to the other. No more shuffling forwards, instead it's the sideways momentum of a pregnant duck-waddle which propels me ahead.

Disgusted with my lack of progress, I retreat back to my bed. My walk confirms it, I've lost more of my faculties, my abilities ... no, not lost, had them taken away, stolen.

This thought stays with me, as visiting time approaches and the ghouls and rats creep around the ward, to menace me. I prepare myself for my visitors, who'll be full of news or want to share thoughts about my health and my future, or distract me with conversations of the past or, worse, their present, an outside, living present that I seem to be denied now my own clock has stopped. Either way, getting through it will be a struggle as I try to claw back my own thoughts and reminiscences from that thief of my soul, try to retrieve those memories that I had not finished with, my fledgling ideas, opinions, prospects and plans which were not yet fully formed before being stolen away. Oh how wicked, that little thief of the night Viral Encephalitis is. Worse still, how can I explain this, to my visitors, who are here to cheer me up?

#

It's another day, another visiting time, yet today I'm so tired it doesn't seem to matter that I don't remember what came before or what is happening now. Nothing really matters.

#

The big D is cropping up in conversations again: discharge. The word confuses me, as I think they are finally going to deal with the incontinence. But no, that's not an issue for them, someone's decided that's a trivial issue which, whilst it encumbers me, does not make it incumbent on the hospital to keep me, to help me; they want to discharge me, in all my filth and failing glory. Once again the conversations seem to be about me, rather than with me, so again it's decided. My discharge is conditional that I stay with Sam and her family for "a fortnight's recovery". This time the doctors and nurses are emphatic with their instructions that I must get lots of rest. For my family, handed the responsibility for the care of this person suffering with a brain injury with all the aplomb and speed of a relay baton, this is the extent of the hospital advice and support offered. For myself, I feel admonished ... I've been resting, for the last two months, but look at me ... will you just look at me?

#

Just before I'm discharged, my brother comes to visit. He's an acupuncturist by profession and he has a keen interest in nutrition. He suggests that I should start juicing and is full of advice about which juicer I should use, the best properties of which fruits and vegetables, what to use and of course what to avoid. Most of the information washes over me, so he helpfully writes down the make and model of his suggested machine, which he feels is more geared towards juicing for medical purposes, so that I can make use of it later. I've always tried to enjoy something of a clean diet particularly since being under Dr. Shen, so I'm not unfamiliar with juicing itself, I'm just familiar with a different kind of juicer. Of course the irony is that even my old juicer will be a re-learning curve, so I may just as well start over. Juicing seems to makes sense to me, as a means to helping my recovery.

And I don't just mean in terms of nutritional benefits. As my brother talks about it, although the detail of what's involved sounds like more faff than I have the energy for currently, I understand that it will probably be good for me and everything I am still trying to do to recover my everyday independence and those taken-for-granted skills, such as reading and writing. Juicing, as I discover, has several facets that should help me, involving shopping for fresh produce, preparing ingredients and following recipes. From where I am now, this sounds like an awful lot of hard work, but an appropriate challenge for someone like me, whoever I might be. It might also give me a sense of purpose. I might feel perky at the thought of this, if, in itself, it didn't all feel like quite so much of an uphill struggle.

But, slowly, slowly, I am ready to be discharged again, almost at the end of the second full month and another whole month since being re-admitted. It's now March 17th, St Patrick's Day. This seems an auspicious date, for this Irish lady, to leave the hospital for what we all hope is the last time, with the reminders from the staff for "lots of rest" and the fact that "this will take time" swirling in the storm of my ears.

6. A "Fortnight's Recovery"

I'm cosy in the bedroom, here at Sam's house. Sam and Simon have worked hard to get it ready for me – they've even moved a wardrobe over from my own house. Although a pain for them to go to such effort for just a fortnight, it's a lovely gesture to help me feel more at home. As a result, after the mayhem of hospital, with pyjamas and underwear going backwards and forwards for laundry, I can have the pleasure of wearing my own clothes, which can be kept neat and creaseless in the wardrobe.

In fact, the only thing in the room which isn't neat and creaseless is me. I'm prone in this bed, with limbs of jelly – no strength or substance at all, a wrinkled bundle of fatigue and confusion. I've been allowed home, but I'm not at home, I'm "recovering" but I feel worse now than the first time I was discharged, last month. Although I don't remember what happened or why I was taken back into hospital, I remember how my body felt and it wasn't like this.

Beyond the wall, in the bedroom next door, I hear the baby start to cry, proper heart-rending baby sobs. It must be loud, if I can hear it through the walls. I can feel it too, the desperation behind it and it strikes a chord with me, causing real toddler tears of my own to start falling. In part it seems that I'm crying for no other reason other than the fact the baby girl I adore is crying, but I know too that it's because I'm afraid, I fear for her.

The constant fear of passing a virus on to anyone, but especially to my little granddaughter is heightened by this, my new proximity to her. The doctors have assured me that this won't happen – Encephalitis is not a transmissible condition, but what about the original infection … I must have caught it from somewhere? Oh my God, it just terrifies me that it could be possible. My own children are adults; they would have some chance of fighting it but a tiny baby, premature at birth, what chance would she have? The thought won't let my head rest so, overwhelmed with fear, I can't stop the tears.

This is what I mean. Last time I was here, in this very bedroom, I was hopeful in my steps to recovery but now I seem to have less about me cognitively … I'm scared and miserable and I still just want to sleep, except I fear that too.

#

A different routine is kicking in, largely organised around my medications. The hospital discharge came with copious prescriptions which Sam dutifully fetched from the pharmacy. From my "previous life" of acupuncture and herbs to remedy my body, I now take prescribed pharmaceuticals as the advocated cornerstones of a possible and ongoing recovery.

The trouble is, I'm just not feeling the benefit from them and I'm hideously confused (as well as painfully slow) when it comes to sorting the dosage and timings of when to take them and which ones should be taken before or with food, so with this comes another dispiriting episode of role–reversal, as Sam takes over the dispensing of my medicine, until I'm well enough to do it myself. Kindly, she makes me a chart to help me follow the medication routine and keep track:

1. Prednisolone 8 X 5mg with or after food
2. Lansoprazole-Gastro Resistant X 1Tablet
3. Allercalm 1 Tablet-as required 4 hourly
4. Paracetamol X 2 –as required
5. Zoplicone x 1tablet before bed.
6. Alendrolic acid

Something called Chlorphenamine and other meds also appear periodically and, with the shrug of a moody teenager, I state my absence of any knowledge about what they're for, what they do. However, it turns out that these are all medications that I know about, apparently, easily solved with an "of course you remember", but of course, I don't.

Sam brings the chart she's made up to my room. It has spaces for morning, lunch, tea and bed times, all ready to be ticked, so that I can follow them. She suggests I should put it up on the wall, so that I can keep track, so that I won't forget.

My eyes flit from her face to the chart and back again. She starts bustling about the room and I feel a surprising surge of anger, fuelled by a sense of total inadequacy and, as she's the only person around, she receives the vent of my frustration. I tell her not to make me one of her projects, my thoughts out there before I have a chance to vet them for any kind of mis-interpretation or offence, or even realise that they may need to be vetted. I can tell she's biting her tongue as she leaves the room.

#

Project or not, a routine for the meds is established and, just as it bore the brunt of the insidious visit of the thief, my body now copes with the pharmaceutical remedies to allegedly help it to repair. It doesn't take long for the steroids to make their presence felt. I catch sight of myself in the mirror, a freak with a full-moon face and it's clear to me that I've not just lost parts of my brain, many of my skills and simple bodily functions, my look has also changed into something I don't recognise. I'm definitely not myself, inside or out.

Like the thief before them, the steroids also play havoc with my system. I go from being exhausted in my bed to being on energy over-drive. I think I'm what you'd call 'high'. I hardly sleep, but need to keep incessantly busy. I'm desperate to write and I grab my laptop or scraps of paper and scribble incessantly - lists, plans and reminders. It's vital that I try to share what seems to be trapped inside me, but of course my toddler scrawls are indecipherable. Still, it's important to keep track of these, as well as my letters from the hospital, work letters, financial correspondence and bank statements, so I create piles of my very important papers, VIPs if you will. Unhappily though, despite my diligence to my paperwork, my industrious shuffling of papers from one pile to another, I keep losing important letters, losing track of what I'm doing: I don't know what's where or why, including myself.

As a distraction, I decide to make the most of the freedom of being 'at home' or at least out of hospital, by phoning my friends both for the joy of contact with the outside world and in the hope of support. It turns out that this too is unsatisfactory therapy. For one thing I can't hear them properly, even with the phone on speaker and for another, I just want to talk, get the words out before they are lost from me, all of which makes for effusive, one-sided conversations at best. My friends and family appear to get bored of this long before I do and definitely before I even notice.

#

My early morning routine is the high-spot of my day, for a short while at least. Evie is now 10 months old and Sam brings her into my room every morning, to say good-morning and have a cuddle, my domestic equivalent of happy hour. Whilst her mum has a peaceful shower or gets on with the millions of chores each day presents to the working mum of a small child, I snuggle the baby, kissing and stroking the fine down of her tender baby head as she generally snoozes beside me. I feel useful and unafraid, for a short while.

And it is a short while, for after happy hour comes cold sweat time as my joyful moment soon passes to the darker side of my mind and my fears press the baby's vulnerability upon me. I never snooze with her because I am afraid for her, afraid of letting her fall. This rational fear morphs and shifts, taking root in some spot of complete irrationality, somewhere between my heart and my mind. I see myself walking into walls with her in my arms, I see her clawed, scratched and hurt by an assailant unknown, I see her touching the sharp blades of the juicer. My heart's pounding as I'm faced with my own inability to protect her. Me, her own grandmother.

I'm aware of an irony. This illness has catapulted my body into an old age, but my mind into some strange infancy, where I can't even look after myself, let alone protect this precious little being. Despite the doctors' assurances about the virus, I'm continually tormented by the idea that the thief might come for Evie too. I have no more chance of escaping the notion than I did of escaping the thief itself, way back in January.

#

Just like the hospital, although on a more flexible schedule, I have visitors. I look forward to this, as much as the drugs and fuddle allow me to. Dave, my counselling manager comes to see me. As he was probably one of the last people to see me as my old self, there's some comfort in just being able to share with him the horrors of this new person I've become. What's more, he's a dedicated, professional listener, so I don't hold back before sharing my thoughts, not that I really try generally, of course.

So, whilst Dave sits there I share the grim kaleidoscope of what the drugs are doing to my head and the fact that this whole illness, along with the medication to support this supposed recovery, have changed me into someone else, someone I would rather not be! I share the details of my dreams and those hideous waking nightmares which still terrify me, these images of what is happening do not belong to me, I would never hurt anyone yet I see falls, I see myself walking into walls whilst carrying a child, knives doing endless damage, accidents with the bloody juicer - hands getting caught. I explain that I'm trapped, caught between logical thinking and the fears of my heart and soul, from which the drugs offer no release but instead some warped exaggeration. And for his part, Dave listens.

#

We decide it's time for a little excursion, Sam and I. She needs to go to the chemist for some supplies for baby Evie and I have a prescription to collect, so this seems to be as good a first outing for me as any. Instantly I feel the same mix of excitement and fear as when I was discharged from the hospital on that first occasion – I'm moving out of a comfort zone, which terrifies me, but moving on a step in my recovery, which I crave.

After much preparation and bundling up in warm clothes against what's proving to be a chilly spring, both myself and baby Evie are ready for the outing. Being out in the car for pleasure is almost a shock to the system, I think I've forgotten that there's a whole world out there, after my prolonged periods inside or perfunctory ferrying to appointments. The outside world rushes past me at a pace as terrifying as a fairground ride, whilst I cling on to the door handle. I'm going to like the spring and getting out more, I think, but not in the car.

Inside the chemist shop it's bright and colourful – so much colour. Sam wanders off to make her purchases whilst I look around in wonderment. There are so many things I love which I had forgotten about, not my nail varnish of course but lipsticks, for instance, with their cheering tones and alluring sheens, lined up like jewels in their racks. I know I'm taking a long time looking at them, but they seem amazing to me, I'm entranced. Finally, I'm reminded about the prescription so I go to the counter to get it. The pharmacist is chatty and helpful about the medications and my difficulties. She suggests a plastic dispensing box with the days of the week on it, to help me to be independent and organised. It has to be said, it's an awful looking box, but it seems practical and useful and, as she's being very kind and attentive, I pay her for the box, as well as my prescriptions.

So, now we're back at Sam's, we set the box up for the coming week, Sam's nimble fingers making short work of the task, job done. She bobs off to see to the baby and I stay here, alone, contemplating the box which has the dubious honour of being the first thing I've bought, on my first outing, since going into hospital two months ago. I don't look at it for long. It disgusts me. I want to throw it at the wall. I don't know why I bought it, I don't deserve it; I wish I'd bought a lipstick. What I really deserve is a new lipstick.

#

The minutes and hours of my "fortnight's recovery" tick slowly by. My family are patient with me as I take so much time and need so much help – getting down the stairs is arduous and slow, getting to the car for appointments and then having to get out again, up and down, in and out, all of those movements I've spent my whole life taking for granted now need planning and permission from my sore brain before the muscles can follow through with any action, any purpose.

After the first week, for the most part, I am in the house on my own as Sam's maternity leave has now finished and she's returned to work three days each week. Being alone in the house brings another role-reversal, in the form of a whole set of instructions and restrictions, like a teenager trusted with the run of the house and no babysitter. I agree readily to them, all the while scared of other unknowns that we might not have thought about:

* The iron and the cooker are off-limits; in case I forget they're on and leave them unattended.
* I mustn't use the bath while alone.
* I should carry my mobile at all times, in case I need to summon help.

For me, this is the worst of all. Sam gives me a neck purse, black with an elephant in beads and sequins on it, from some far flung holiday she took in the past. When I don't have a pocket (which seems to be quite often) I have to wear the purse around my neck, with my phone inside.

It's true to say that I hate this elephant. It's a parody of my situation, of Viral Encephalitis itself. Elephants never forget right? Yet here I am, memory almost wiped clean by the virus and having to make myself remember to wear the purse, for carrying the mobile, for contacting the help, because I'm not really safe on my own – I have inabilities and considerable limitations, thanks to both the illness and the drugs. Elephants are scared by mice, right? And here I am again, terrified by the plagues of rats which sneak around my brain and peripheral vision. The Encephalitis is the elephant in the room, the weight of which I have to bear around my neck.

I want to object to the restrictions, break the rules, yet I know they're necessary and what's more, I'm too terrified not to follow them. When you realise that everything is still the same, it's only you who has changed, it's very scary to have to try to do what's necessary to make it better. It's scary not only because I have no idea what will make it better but also because I'm finding it so hard to cope - there's no one around who understands how I feel. I know I'm lucky to have friends who are counsellors and apparently I haven't been shy with subjecting Dave to the nasty end of everything that ails and fails me; but this? This I have to work on alone ... and I do feel very much alone.

#

As the days without Sam's presence stretch themselves menacingly in front of me, I'm trying to establish a kind of routine. To start with, I've just stayed in my room, too scared to go downstairs, afraid, afraid of everything: of using the stairs; of leaving something switched on; of leaving the door unlocked. But this fear is getting me nowhere, in all senses, so I have to try harder, I know I have to try harder, not least because it's so tedious up here. I can't sleep, can't read or write, can't use my hands properly for any kind of crafting amusement. I am lonely and I am bored. In short, I am plain miserable.

#

I'm downstairs today. On my own I manage the stairs by sitting down and bumping my way down on my bottom. This hurts my head more than it hurts my bum, but it's safer than walking and possibly falling. However, the effect of the bumping on the incontinence is not up for discussion. Suffice it to say that once I land safely, my next stop is the downstairs cloakroom.

From here, my time downstairs is spent facing my fears, in all of their cunning guises of constant shadows and lights which I catch flitting and flickering from the corners of my eyes. I can feel a presence and I know that someone is standing behind me and whichever way I look, at the edge of my vision I see the movement of shadows and the menacing reflections of encroaching colours. Was that a face? An arm passing an open door? Meanwhile, rats and mice flit from place to place, they have followed me here from the hospital. No-one else sees them but I see them all the time, behind cushions, behind curtains; watching, waiting.

I try to be purposeful, despite them. I can't do the really useful things for Sam, like the laundry and ironing, or preparing the meal, but I can try the menial jobs, like dusting and tidying and, as the weather improves, it would be nice to get out into the back garden. The back door is easier to lock and I can leave it open whilst I'm outside without fear of it slamming shut on me. In the meantime, I shuffle around, trying to get my confidence back and not catch the eyes of the ghouls.

#

One particular challenge I have set myself, is the juicer. After my brother's advice, I ordered the specified machine which duly arrived here, at Sam's, a few days after I did. I regard this juicer with suspicion, representing as it does both conflicts and challenges to me.

The conflicts lie within the fact that my brother's suggested that juicing will benefit my health ... scrap that, what health? My recovery, then. I'm inclined to believe him, not only because he knows what he's talking about professionally and is personally concerned for my well-being, but also of course based on my previous success with acupuncture, using herbs and my time with Dr. Shen; I believe in the benefits of such remedies, even if I can no longer remember why I believe.

However, my perception of these benefits conflicts gravely with my warped perceptions of the juicer as an instrument of harm, courtesy of my waking nightmares of its blades, it's ability to chop and slice with clinical precision and surgical autonomy to innocent flesh. This is where my nightmares, daymares and fearful hallucinations clearly affect my logic. This is a masticating juicer, which has no blades, just tiny teeth – vicious no doubt but well protected. There's no harm here for myself or the little one, yet to my subconscious fears it's still an instrument of violence.

And the challenges? Juicing, I discover, presents a three-fold challenge to me: I have to follow a recipe, which means I have to make a shopping list, legibly. I also have to assemble the machine each time, do the juicing and then disassemble and carefully wash the relevant parts. All of these actions present important, practical challenges in themselves but also a greater experience of practice and repeat, practice and repeat. This strikes me as important therapy in itself and, as much as "of course you remember" has become a mantra which reflects my inabilities, "practice and repeat" is becoming something of my personal retort, reflecting my slow progress in some ways but also my ability and willingness to try.

#

Meanwhile, the calendar turns to April and accordingly, my "fortnight's recovery" is up. But it isn't, is it? One look at me, with my racked body and moon face, one conversation with me, with my unfinished sentences, lost words and forthright candour, is enough to show anyone that my "self" is still lost and within that context, recovery hasn't even begun.

Despite all the medication, my immune system is shot and my throat seems to be in a constant flare. I see the GP for antibiotics and we end up having a longer chat, about how I *really* am. He's so kind to me that I cry, once again sobbing for what I am now, at the cost of what I am no longer.

I tell him that I've been in touch with the Encephalitis Society and he agrees that an Encephalitis support group might be helpful and I readily agree, waiting for him to offer more information, to forge the link for me with others who have struggled with Viral Encephalitis (VE), to access support and rehabilitation contacts. Even as I wait for him to offer a referral, he shrugs off the suggestion: in truth, he doesn't actually know of any support local groups, instead the best he can offer is that he still finds it hard himself to believe that I've had Encephalitis and that, all being well, I "should feel better by Christmas". His words hit me, a side-swipe of disbelief as my scrambled brain tries to time-line this in the context of the hospital's cursory adieu of a "fortnight's recovery". We're in April ... Christmas is months away! I can do nothing but start sobbing anew and for his part, the GP can do nothing but gently suggest that I check with the neurologist.

#

I'm told that, because I have an Acquired Brain Injury (ABI), I should report my condition to the Driver and Vehicle Licensing Agency (DVLA). So this is what I do. Or actually I don't, at least not for a while, because it seems impossible to get through to them on the phone. Along with the juicing, it has become a daily mission to try to get through, which adds a strange can-do sense of purpose to my days, ironic considering the fact I'm trying to inform them of what I can't do. I call them several times without success, but finally get through to customer services on the very day that the officially trained helpers are on strike.

"I'm sorry, I can't help you," says the person manning the phones. I guess there's more than a little truth in that.

Eventually I receive the necessary form, which Sam helps me to go through. There are several possible options and choices and I feel scared to commit myself, partly because I'm still confused and can't track time very well and partly from having been so unknowing and innocent of the inset of the Encephalitis, I fight shy of making decisions which smack of a future as yet unknown, of a full recovery as yet inconceivable.

Sam advises me to choose the medical assessment option, as apparently this way I won't have to re-take my driving test to resume driving, whenever that might be. I'm not sure which fills me with the most horror, the idea of being behind the wheel and in control of a car or the thought of having to re-take my driving test. In the event, I let Sam take the driving seat in the discussion and I opt for the medical assessment which can come later on. Much later on, I suspect.

#

There's a palpable tension in the house and I'm painfully aware that my presence is its source. That fortnight's recovery, so often mentioned in the hospital, is not just a time-line for me and my recovery from VE, but also suggested an expectation for my daughter and her family, their own rough guide of how long they might expect to have mother, mother-in-law and grandmother (complete now with grandmotherly walking sticks and incontinence pads) in their home. Not stressful enough? Well add to that the physical and mental illness on my part, along with the pressures on a young working family with their tiny, very premature baby and possibly some postnatal depression too and you have, to say the least, a difficult situation for anyone to be in.

Alongside all this is that role change, the one I don't like and that Sam didn't necessarily bargain for. In these past few weeks she's had to become my parent and I, her child. Part of the problem with this is that I'm hideously aware that I'm supposed to be the parent, yet I don't seem to have any parental status, much less abilities.

I'm in my room contemplating this and what to do about it when, with the true force of a high drama, cinematic flashback, I recall myself back in the hospital, telling the charming consultant that he could not let me die as my children only had me, a sole parent. I've been their only parent, by my choice, for so long and could not let them down, but the irony is of course overwhelming: I have let them down, by being so sick and needing all of this help and attention. I've always been the strong one and it would be allowing the thief to have all of me if I died, yet inside I've also been craving to be allowed the easy way out. With a shock, I realise that I haven't received any of those things my confused wish-list demanded: I'm alive, but no longer a parent in the functional sense of the word. The baby starts crying from her crib in the bedroom next door, her tears for her mummy. It's not long before mine start again also, for the mummy missing to me too.

#

We're out in the car, Sam driving, on our way to the farm shop to get some fresh vegetables for my juicing. The plan is for her to nip into Tesco and then we'll go on to the farm shop. It's a pleasant morning although the outing brings a paradox: I'm glad to be getting some fresh veg and extras for my juicing, but I'm not too happy to be in the car, it continues to terrify me and I still feel strange in the passenger seat. In the early days of my business, I did a lot of driving between clients and suppliers, so the thoughts and reactions of a driver are deeply ingrained. As such, I view the scenery with my keen driver's eyes, as alert as I can be without my licence or, indeed, the full faculties required to drive myself. I wonder how I managed to drive all those miles each week for work, being behind the wheel seems to require so much attention and concentration.

As we pull out of Tesco, I comment to Sam about another driver who I think has been waiting for her: "I think she was letting you go" I tell her.

No sooner are the words out of my mouth like a red rag, than the bull of her pent up stress begins its full nostril flare, stamping foot and run up. A tirade rushes from Sam's lips, nothing to do with my back-seat driving, but everything to do with my front-seat living; the apparent prioritising of my own needs over everyone else's.

I'm stunned ... I'm the one who's sick, look at what happened to me, will you just look at what happened to me? My own words can't come quick enough to point this out. "Why should you need anything, you're not sick?" I cry. I just cannot understand her argument or her anger.

We arrive at the farm shop, our mutual resentment waving like a banner from the car. Sam shouts at me that I'm angry and, to be honest, I don't understand this as a point of argument either; of course I'm angry, angry doesn't even begin to describe this person who is not herself, who hasn't got a clue what she's doing or what's going to happen, most of the time. I get up angry and I go to bed scared, if my emotions change to anything positive in between then it's been a good day as far as I'm concerned. Angry? I'm bloody furious and who would expect otherwise?

It's not until much later that I realise that our role-reversals have contributed to, and had a much bigger effect on, the tension in the house than I had thought. As Sam's parent, I've always known that she needs to have a row to get things off her chest. That's just her way. Today's argument means that not only am I now unable to recognise the child I should know, but I've also failed to recognise that her reaction is an angry response, or some kind of projection of anger over her own loss of the mother she knew. Caught in our own cross-fire, I can see that there are injuries on both sides, wounds which, if we're not careful, will take a long time to heal.

7. "Like It or Lump It"

Conversations are starting to take a turn towards the future, my future. Sam suggests that we talk about it and as soon as the proposal is out there my sister Frances, who has come to visit me, is quick to notice how personal and emotional the subject is. She asks me if I would like her to be around for the conversation, or if I'd prefer her not to be. When I tell her that I'd like her to sit in on it, Sam suggests that we talk later in the evening, when her husband too can be present.

And so, once the baby is in bed, we have our chat about my future. However, instead of a dialogue, an exchange, I feel bombarded with questions which I just don't know the answers to: will I be able to live independently? Will I be in danger of falling? The stairs - here, back home, anywhere - will I be able to manage without falling down them? Do I want to live with other people?

Confused, I offer to try to find out about what support might be available to me, to help me to live independently, but this seems to come across as something of a slight. That's not how I mean it, I'm just being practical. This is me we're talking about, isn't it? What *I* need? And it doesn't come without a cost to me, this valiant suggestion of mine. Don't they realise that I hate having to ask for help? That nowadays I spend most occasions going down the stairs on my bottom, my poor, sore bottom, rather than ask for help?

The truth is, the conversation's made a subtle turn into who's had, and indeed is still having, the hardest time. So now, instead of discussing the future, I'm feeling caught in a point-scoring match and some strange push-pull situation - depend on me, try to be independent; we're here to help, but help yourself, for goodness sake. Confusion is taking over. It's hard for me being poorly, living with them; it's hard for them, living with me, looking after me, being responsible for me ... I do realise that, but it's not my fault, don't they see? I start to feel emotional which is the worst possible thing when I need to be able to think rationally about my situation, what my next move should be, what I'm likely to need help with and, crucially, when I'm going to be able to move on.

Eventually, my son-in-law sums up my options by telling me that I'm in a "like it or lump it situation." Although I know he's well meaning, his words strike me as cruel, like a swift kick to a helpless kitten. I can't take my eyes off him as my insides threaten to explode, spill over the boundaries of my own resilience.

"With due respect, Simon, I am not your mother … and nobody tells me to like it or lump it!" the words are out of my mouth as I think them and it's now impossible not to cry, my eyes and heart just leaking their hurt and betraying my vulnerability despite my feisty words. The realisation that they think they have no choice but to have me here, which of course they insisted on, is too much. Other arrangements could have been made …in fact, they should have been made; I should have been in rehab. This shouldn't be happening to any of us, not them, least of all me. This crying is exhausting but I can't stop it; I have no more control over my tears than I do over any other aspect of my situation. No, I don't like it but I'll be darned if I'll lump it either and what's more, it's too soon, far too soon to be told that these are my options in life. I want to go home, but more than that, I want to be well enough to go home.

#

I'm at a loss, and it's all about my loss.

#

As April drags on, I'm desperate to extend my repertoire of can-do tasks. If nothing else, the "like it or lump it" comment, driven possibly by their own fears for my future, motivates me to change my situation, to manage and to get better.

I constantly write … well, scribble but no matter how much I commit to paper, I can't ever convey the feelings of fear, desperation and complete uselessness that just churn away inside of me, like a volcano waiting to erupt. I don't know if this is because I've lost the right words or if there just aren't the words for it. I'm surrounded by blank sheets of paper just as I'm surrounded by an empty, lonely pain which I just can't shift.

Where I can't find words, I try to focus my mind on numbers. I'm spending hours with my personal accounts and I catch the word "obsessed" being uttered from time to time. But, whatever anyone else thinks, I'm thankful that I can focus, for longer spells, on this. I check my personal accounts, watch my withdrawals and double-check my spending, penny by penny, pound by pound. I've become pedantic about paying what I owe and I fret constantly about cash flow and debt. The more I fret, the more I'm drawn back to my accounts, to try to keep up with things.

Flushed with my relative success at focusing on the numbers, keeping my own accounts going, and my ongoing wish to fill the void of my own existence with practical tasks, I have the startling realisation about the next step in my recovery: I'm going to try getting back to the business. The thought isn't a scary one, in fact it's feeling like one of my better ideas lately.

Sam and one of my colleagues, Lorraine, have been keeping things afloat whilst I've been ill and I'm so grateful that, now I feel ready, I'm convinced I should try to relieve them of some of the stress of it. Of course, Sam's been familiar with the business since her teenage years, when she used to help me occasionally, so she's been handling the stock. Lorraine has worked part time for me for some years in accounts and is used to doing the invoicing, so between them they've done a really good job of keeping it going. For my part, I can't begin to explain how much I appreciate their efforts, although I do try.

I tell Sam about my plan and she offers to drive me in, next time she's going to the office and so, I start my road not just towards recovery, but back towards business. Lorraine is of course very pleased to see me and we spend much of my first visit catching up. She tells me that some of the suppliers had been very helpful with regards to ordering stock, a task that neither she nor Sam have been particularly familiar with and once again I'm humbled by people's willingness to try to help, even though I was in my darkest hours of neither knowing, or caring less, at the time.

After our catch up though, it's clear that Sam and Lorraine have their own, newly established routine, within which I lurk on the periphery, not really fitting. I try to carry out a few menial tasks, filing, sorting, checking whilst they chat away as if I'm not there. My bubble of being back in the business does not burst as such, but instead deflates, slowly, like a forgotten balloon once a celebration is over. I'm not included in their conversations or referred to with respect for the woman I used to be, the owner of the business, who I am or, in fact, any of the things I am to them: mother, employer, friend and colleague. It might be that they are trying to "normalise" the situation for my benefit I suppose but, as I bring a sheaf of statements home to fold and envelope, a job that I've paid someone else to do in the past, my situation feels nothing like good and definitely not as helpful to my recovery as I had hoped. It appears I'm not back in the driving seat, I'm still very much a passenger.

#

"It's good to see you looking so much better." The GP announces this to me with absolute sincerity, then settles back in his chair to smile at me encouragingly.

Every muscle in me has become taut as if something within is about to pop. I feel something close to a very bad temper start to boil up from somewhere deep inside me and I find myself fighting not to just scream at him. I mean, if I can't get my GP to understand that the external achievements he sees are not the whole of me improving, then how am I going to get anyone else to understand it?

It's actually quite easy to look a bit better ... and I don't just mean by comparison, because I looked so ghastly before that anything is an improvement. Part of the apparent "wellness" comes from the simple fact that I can now mostly (albeit slowly and carefully) take care of my own toilette and necessities of personal grooming; that is, run a brush through my own hair, which I've been keeping mercifully short as I can't even hold a hair dryer. But a brush, yes, I can manage that, for goodness sake. Meanwhile, the juicing has helped perk up my tired complexion and of course the infernal steroids give me the chubby, round face associated with a picture of health. But that's all it is, a picture, an image, an illusion.

What lies beneath all this though, is a head, brain, mind – call it what you will - which seem to just do its own thing. I'm assured that I'm behaving normally but I don't feel normal - my writing is poor, my figures mixed up. My mobility is limited, I have no control over my bodily eliminations, so I have no independence and little dignity. Yet, the worst challenge of each day isn't even to do with dealing with all of that ... it's to do with everyone else and the fact that people seem completely unable to comprehend what VE is, the damage it does and the changes it causes to people. And more than that, not even its effect on 'people' in the generic, but to a person in the individual, a person like me.

However, if I speak my mind on this fact I'm told that I should be grateful that I am not worse: "you could have cancer, or be in a coma or a wheelchair."

"I am grateful." I trot out my standard reply, usually through gritted teeth. Yet every night, with silent prayers, I show my gratitude by appealing to God that if I'm not going to get better, then why not just take me? Of course, the truly grateful part of me does want to stay, just not like this.

Trying to keep my voice and temper in check, I try to explain to the GP that it's not about how I look: my look doesn't reflect how I am, how I feel. His answer is that I must rest. Rest, rest, rest. He tells me to forget work, the one thing which focuses me on being at least, in part, recovered.

I guess that's told me, so I move the conversation to supplements: what should I take to aid my brain recovery? "Forget about that," he repeats. "Get plenty of rest, think positively and you should feel better by the end of the year."

I'm aghast once more. Where does this "end of the year" business keep coming from? It's April, the end of the year is eight months from now! He must be mistaken, it cannot take me that long to get better. Rest, rest, rest for eight months more? I'm reminded again of my instructions on leaving the hospital, the need for "lots of rest" and the disclaimer that this will "take time". I assumed that the time they were talking about was the couple of weeks they'd insisted I spend at Sam's house. I thought I understood it all, that in that couple of weeks I was going to make a full recovery.

It seems I was wrong and the GP, with his "end of the year" is more likely to be right. I feel incapable of thinking any more about this, much less reacting to it. My mind switches to an empty abyss as my GP continues to reassure me that what I'm experiencing is all part of my condition and that I can always go back to the neurologist.

But here-in lies another problem. It's not just about the Emperor's new clothes (or grandmother's steroid face) of looking 'better' it's also about the confusion over who has that overall view of what "normal" or "progress" looks like in this post-VE phase. To that end, these numerous medical appointments aren't helping as each time I'm referred to another department or the neurologist, the only thing they seem to concur over is the idea that I should "rest, rest, rest."

What no-one seems to understand is that resting is never going to be an option for me. Sure, I can sit for ten minutes here or there but going for a lie down is a no-no, thanks mostly to my newly-established fear of sleep, borne from my last experience of sleeping, where I did not choose to sleep for so long and I did not wake up as I would have wanted to … in truth, waking up as another person entirely.

So each time I'm supposed to be resting I fear, subconsciously, instinctively, that I am not going to waken or that whilst I'm sleeping the thief will make a visit and I will find myself awakening with even less faculties and abilities. So it is, I cannot take the risk. I push myself on, endlessly on, many days awake by 5am, ready to start another full day of trying to recover, trying to regain my old self. Often I'm awakened by my own tears, which spring forth even as I try to "rest."

Alternatively, I find myself starting to cry as soon as I waken. In the small, lonely hours when this occurs, I allow myself this moment, for this is the time when I don't have to stop myself or be told "think of all you have achieved and stop thinking about what you can't do." Deep down I guess that I am really crying for all that I have lost, my abilities, my personality, my confidence and of course my independence. I'm a shadow of the person I used to be and I mourn her loss, even as I sleep.

And the galling thing is that this moment, this very split second when all these thoughts - my passionate explanation of the trauma associated with resting and the problems with existing in my post-VE state - run through my head, turns out to be the one time my thoughts just can't spring forth, cannot be shared regardless with the GP, the GP who thinks I'm looking better. Instead, I accept my repeat prescription, my revised timeline for recovery and advice to return to the neurologist and quietly, with as much dignity as my sticks and padded rear will allow, exit his room.

8. On Encephalitis

Although my illness has shown up many new, strange aspects to my life, my self, one of the weirdest things which has stayed with me is the fact that, even once finally diagnosed, I could get neither my tongue nor my head around what was wrong with me. When I came round in any kind of coherent, sitting up way, or responded to others, I could not say the word 'Encephalitis' or remember what was wrong with me; I just knew that I was sick in hospital.

Mind you, later on I still can't get my head around "Autoimmune Viral Encephalitis"[(1)] because I don't have a clue what it is, although I'm living proof of what it does. Whilst I know the inner sanctum of my self has been stripped bare by a thief in the night, this explanation for the person I now am isn't present in the careful and repetitive explanations from the medical staff, including the various nurses, consultants and GPs who are all part of my regular care.

They have to repeat their explanations or I have to try to be in some kind of earshot range as they explain to my children because, of course, I don't really remember from day to day what they've said about it, let alone the why and how of the ways I've been so affected by it. The non-scientific but suitably metaphoric spectre of the thief is the only explanation that I can retain, or at least is the only one which seems to make any sense to me, to lie just within the grasp of my understanding.

#

It's not until April 2008, during my "fortnight's recovery" at Sam's when I have, what is for me, a real turning point. Sam tells me there is an Encephalitis Society and, despite my struggles with hearing on the phone, I call them. The man I speak with is so kind to me and extremely helpful that I'm taken aback, without being really sure why. We chat for a while and he agrees to send me information about the condition, rehabilitation and the society's work and outreach, but this isn't what really pleases me. The thing is, as we're talking, I'm aware that what I'm experiencing is a warm glow of acceptance from this man, a perfect stranger. Finally, someone gets it; someone understands what's happened to me, understands what it means, what I'm left with, this bizarre combination of the old and the new.

I'm taken aback though, when he suggests that I speak again to the hospital and get another appointment with the neurologist. He seems to think that this is vital for my overall recovery. Confusion muscles in to squash my newly-found comfort. I tell him that I didn't realise that I'd still need to be attending appointments at the hospital as I cheerily try to dismiss the idea.

"I'm going to be better soon," I share brightly. There's a pause at the other end of the phone, before he politely advises me to seek another appointment, all the same.

He's right of course, the lack of significant follow-up from the hospital is adding to the tension over the prolonged and painfully slow pace of my recovery. What I don't realise though is that as part of my discharge some follow-up appointments have already been put in place. So, as I pursue appointments which may or may not have already been made for me – neurology, physiotherapy, hearing, incontinence clinic - confusion reigns supreme. I find myself scrawling endless lists of the questions I want to ask that pop into my head at random times. I have to remember what I need to ask when I get to each of these appointments, this is incredibly important to me.

He also asks about physiotherapy which is, very literally, a sore subject. I received none in the whole time I was in the hospital and my movement and walking are still dire, my balance skewed, my mobility reliant on sticks, which I hate with a passion; I just can't see them as a means to mobility, more a signifier of my limitations. Finally, the physiotherapy department respond to the hospital's requests with a long awaited phone call. The woman is kind and reassures me that I am entitled to therapy, that's the good news. The bad news? It will be hydrotherapy and, naturally, there's a waiting list. Of course I have nothing better to do than continue to wait to get better, especially it seems if I want the assistance to do so. I'd laugh about it, really I would, if I could stop myself crying.

#

Within a few days I duly receive the information from the Encephalitis Society ... a whole pack which lands with a thud of expectation on the doormat. Eager to learn more about my condition and, importantly, my recovery, I try to read it. This, as much as the juicing, becomes a daily and regular challenge. My reading is still so mechanical and my memory so poor, that I approach the same sentence over and over, trying to read it, understand it, absorb it.

Sam seems furious with me, every time she finds me reading "that bloody book again!" The fact is, I'm not reading the book over and over in search of answers, like an obsessive - I'm actually reading the same page for days on end, not only because like a child I've yet to understand and absorb it but also, as someone with a brain injury, I've forgotten which parts I've already read!

Mind you, at least my brain injury gives me an excuse for not really understanding the effects of Encephalitis on my body. Others seem to have far less excuse. Of the GP husband and wife partnership serving most of my needs since I've been discharged, the Mrs. GP is curt and dismissive of my enquiries about my symptoms, my medication and my prognosis for full recovery. Meanwhile, Mr. GP, although sympathetic and genial, "can't believe" I've had Encephalitis (despite the copies of copious hospital notes which now clog my surgery file) and so offers nothing but wonderment at the fact I've lurched into the surgery to sit in front of him. Any questions I raise are either put down to my medication or to the condition itself, which are easily resolvable from his position with a placatory: "talk to the neurologist."

Which I do, of course. The neurologist is more than helpful and is certainly very patient, but of course I don't know the right questions to ask. Right so of course I ask what's on my mind, or my list, but because I can neither understand my own condition nor absorb his replies, I can't make informed responses or even formulate intelligent questions over and above my fall-back position: "when will I be better?" This is *the* question.

In the event, all of the best answers I ever receive are from the Encephalitis Society. Of course I may not like their answers all the time – years to recover? Really? No, not me, I'll be better soon, won't I? After all, they said two weeks at the hospital, didn't they? However, at least I know there's some specialist experience and understanding behind their advice.

#

From the Encephalitis Society I learn that Encephalitis is indeed a syndrome that affects the brain which, when borne of a virus as mine was, comes with all those flu-like symptoms and confusion that I demonstrated without even knowing what was going on. The actual symptoms might vary depending on which part of the brain is under attack (and I later find out much more about this when my incontinence is finally investigated and I'm told I have three brain spots which have been permanently affected). However, any part of the brain under attack in such a way can suffer significant inflammation which has two effects:

* The brain's messages to other parts of the body can become confused and ineffectual; it controls your whole nervous system after all and everything from your personality, physical abilities, memories and emotions to processing, sensory and communication skills can be affected, as well as the fatigue factor!

* The attack and the subsequent inflammation can destroy neurons, vital nerve cells in the brain. In some cases, damaged neurons may be able to repair themselves over time. Alternatively, neurons may be permanently damaged resulting in a permanent disability unless enough healthy neurons remain to try to compensate for those lost, meaning that the brain is working harder to do everything it used to, but with less neurons to do it.

I'm also fascinated to find that my immune system could be so compromised by the Encephalitis that it can end up causing more damage by attacking itself rather than trying to defend the brain against the virus, something which was investigated in my case.

It's no wonder then, that I'm so tired. I read with despair that damaged brain tissue takes much longer to repair than muscles or bones and the Encephalitis Society's literature states exactly what I'm finding: that because I'm relatively 'better' than I was, others expect that I am now fine. But the truth is that such devastation requires a long healing time, significant rest and considerable support, even rehabilitation depending on the extent of the damage and the symptoms.

I learn so much from the Encephalitis Society's literature that I try to get others to read "that bloody book" so that they can understand the illness, understand me. I would strongly support anyone who's recovering from Encephalitis, or supporting someone to rebuild their life after this dreadful illness, to get in touch with the Encephalitis Society in the first instance. It's not just a way of finding out more, it's also a way of realising that you're not alone in both the situation you find yourself in and on the long road that lays ahead, so I've included the contact details for the society at the end of the book.

#

As time moves on, it becomes important to me to become more involved with the Encephalitis Society. This urge, I think, is driven by two significant factors:

* At my worst, I had no one local to talk to. If I'd been diagnosed with cancer, the wonderful local (and national) Macmillan support team would have been available immediately, thank heavens. However, find yourself with a lesser known but completely disabling condition such as Encephalitis and you're on your own in my local area, despite the fact that there are a similar number of cases as some forms of cancer, per year. So, if I could be that person for someone else, someone local, someone scared, someone like me, then surely I should help if I can?
* I believe in paying things back. Having discovered the Encephalitis Society, I hugged their virtual presence to me like a security blanket ... checking their literature to compare my own notes, following their development in raising awareness, painstakingly reading their recommended books, using their advised questions when visiting the GP and neurologist. If I could pay them back for the help they've given me, continue to give me, then of course I want to do so. This also ties into my need to help others suffering from the aftermath of this dreadful condition. I want to pay the support I receive forwards, too.

#

In the fullness of time, I try to become more involved. I slowly move from being a recipient of their newsletters, to being a contributor. Then, as time moves on, far beyond this, the first year of illness, of 'recovery' I find I am able to offer more, to contribute more. By the latter part of 2009, although it takes considerable effort, I volunteer to organise the occasional fundraising coffee morning for the Encephalitis Society. For the very first one of these, I am stricken with anxiety, worrying whether I have thought of everything and literally trying to get my head around the planning: when to shop; when to bake; how to set up?

Of these, baking is a major challenge. I have no confidence about that but I am determined I am going to find out if I am able to. The trouble is, I've already planned it badly because the week of the first event is also my birthday week. I get addled when two things happen close together, they merge in my mind and I'm flustered just by the idea of it all: I genuinely think I will not be able to fit it all in. I just hadn't factored in that I would be out on Thursday evening for a birthday dinner and of course as always happens this is the week that work suddenly becomes very busy. I've also got a lunch booked with the girls on the Friday but kindly they offer to be available afterwards, to give me a hand, so I keep my fingers crossed that all will go well.

In the event, my anxiety eases as the week arrives and with it lots of birthday gifts and cards and a humbling amount of help and support. Despite the fact that Saturday dawns as a very wet, miserable day, I feel surprisingly bright and sunny in myself. As I can't spread the event out into the garden, the house quickly feels packed and buzzing as nearly 40 people come through my front door in the course of the morning. A local boutique, *Who's Wearing What*, join in the fray to add both to the fund raising potential and the crush in my living room, with a rail of wears for sale for my visitors to try. I'm so excited: each person counted is a measure of my success, even in attempting the event, even though we haven't counted up contributions yet. And when we do? £180.72 raised. A small amount in real terms, but for me a big achievement.

#

As a result of my fundraising efforts, I'm invited to the Encephalitis Society's 15th birthday bash at the Canal

Museum in London. I can't explain the surge that comes with this invitation, the excitement of being wanted, appreciated, invited all mixed up with the sheer horror of a trip to London, for a party by the Thames in the closing months of the year ... a direct parallel to my first experience of becoming ill, all that time ago.

I know I'll manage much better with company and support, and the invitation also includes "guest", so I immediately ask Sam if she'll accompany me. Unfortunately she's unable to and so as the saying goes, regretfully declines. Instead, my friend Glenda accepts my invitation to come.

This brings me two things: yes the company and support, but also a resurgence of something I've been so lacking, that shadow of my lost femininity. Now I have that "what shall I wear?" dilemma and, excitingly, someone to share that feeling and the ensuing expedition for a whole new frock with, something which removes several layers of the isolation I usually find myself wrapped up in. Ok, so it's not that I am short of outfits, but nothing feels as it once did, nothing's good on this strange new body, so I decide to buy something new. This full-on shopping quest also provides a useful trial-run for the rigours and exertion of attending the event itself.

And it works, at least for a while, to temper some of my fears, of the sheer effort of something that was once a common practice - of hopping on the train to London. To be so unable to take such an "easy" thing for granted is to once again be confronted with my inabilities and limitations. It's daunting. It not only takes effort to do such activities but also, depending on my day, my mind, my clarity, it also takes extreme effort to be able to say to myself that this, the Encephalitis and what the thief left behind, cannot stop me.

And so, the unstoppable I and the kindly Glenda take the train to London. As the train rushes through the sprawling skirts of the city, I wonder at the things that used to be so familiar but have since, along with various capabilities and memories, been forgotten: the London Eye; the Gherkin; the lights; the speed of the escalator in Charing Cross; the adverts for movies I've never heard of; 30p to go to the loo to spend a penny (because of course I still have all that to see to); the tube to Paddington; the fear of the pacing mass of people walking and even running; at the crush of the crowds who rush at me, by me. I'm swept up with the tide of city transport, with Glenda as my only anchor.

After the trial of train and tube we walk along the canal basin, in the bitter cold, quickly deciding to warm up with a bowl of soup while we wait for the appointed time. The Union, the pub / restaurant we slide into, is busy, heaving with cheerful city folk. The staff are nice and friendly but the noise in my ears is unbelievable – it's just conversation, the hubble, bubble and excitement of others, but it's a roar in my ears, my head. I do what I have always done at conferences and exhibitions, largely out of instinct more than memory: I put the Encephalitis Society's invitation on the table, just as I would have done with a company brochure. When you do this, others going to the same event often say hello, so that you know you'll have a friendly face in the crowds when you get there, but here, today, no one apart from the staff speaks to us, so I guess the other guests are still on their way or are waiting elsewhere.

Of course, I should have guessed that if the pub was "noisy" then the actual event would be pretty overwhelming. With all the sounds associated with a celebration, a party, along with the sights and the physicality involved in taking the special barge trip, before arriving at the canal museum.

However, what's lost to me in a sense of overwhelming noise is recompensed with an atmosphere of complete welcome and understanding. This evening's the first real chance to meet and talk with those who have been there, done that, flailed in the hospital tunic, as well as those who have supported a 'victim'. When I'm not fighting my own senses to be able to participate in conversations, when I'm not totally distracted by being incontinent of my bowel (which is unfortunately up to three times a day at the moment) and of course I've been on my feet a lot today, then, and despite it all, I'm finally able to share my experience with those who understand best.

One lady nods sagely, as I outline that famous "give it until Christmas" advice. She tells me to forget everything I've been told about it taking two years, "why, it's more like four to seven, to recover or to get over it!" she shares. Although I'm a little shocked, I agree with her because it actually makes sense. Yes, we agree that the timeline seems unbelievable but it's not only that, it's also the fact that the illness itself is such a shock to the system that makes the whole thing so very hard to get over, if ever.

It's great also to not be alone over all those little details that come with the illness ... not least the attitudes of others. Along with these very special, and truly compassionate companions I'm able to laugh for the first time at those habits others have which aggravate me so much in daily life: the annoying responses of saying "oh that happens to me" when you share a memory loss, when you've missed an appointment, or spend your time fretting over having to work from a diary to know what on earth it is you're meant to be doing. Yes, it's laughable, we agree and indeed we do laugh, that they have no idea what it is like to have to write a day-to-day list and constantly use a diary – just to stay on top of daily life, especially if you have never done that before. We all agree that this "me too!" sharing is a kindly attempt on others' part to try and normalise a situation for us. Yet, for us, the afflicted, we agree that it feels like not being heard, like having worries just being dismissed as trivial. I've always berated myself for the fact that I find this "oh yes, haven't we all ...?" attitude hugely upsetting, but in my present company I realise the fault isn't necessarily mine. A weight lifts. Yes, my usual angry response reflects an attitude problem, but not of mine, nor even of an attitude towards me, but of a lack of tolerance, a lack of understanding of Encephalitis itself and of even less understanding of how we feel.

Regrettably, Glenda and I have to leave before the event finishes, so we can be sure of not missing our train home. I'm exhausted, senses reeling, but for the first time since being invalided by Encephalitis, I feel the sense of my own validity: I *know* I'm far greater than the sum of unbalanced parts and partial functions the thief has left me with and I know that it's OK for me to acknowledge this. For the first time, in a long time, I experience a shred of acceptance, intrinsic as well as from those kind people I'm now acquainted with.

#

Within a short time, just the following year I'm invited by the Encephalitis Society to apply to be a regional representative. Once again, a sense of validity, long misplaced since my business, my counselling and my choral group singing fell by the wayside in the thief's wake, raises an unexpectedly proud head. I submit my application, which is no mean feat in itself.

I'm elated when, a few weeks after submitting it, I get a call to say I've been selected. This is what I want: to be able to pay it forwards as well as give something back. I eagerly reach for my diary as they ask me to come for training in April. My diary, usually my stalwart advisor, delivers a crushing blow: the date of the training weekend is rattled off, despite my "pardon, please can you repeat that?" down the phone. It's worse than being unable to hear them, I'm unable to attend: the date is already filled in my diary, with events and appointments, reminders of my circuit of illness and wellness, ongoing recovery. I have to turn down this training opportunity.

"Don't worry," the lady on the phone says brightly. "I'll give you the dates for next year and put you in for those." So there I am, on a waiting list once more, for the one training weekend running in the whole year; instead of waiting for help, I'm now waiting *to* help.

Personal note

It should be noted that the term noted (1) Autoimmune Viral Encephalitis, as used by the physicians when discussing my condition, is the formal denotation of the condition, such as used in medical journals. It's possible that the form of my Viral Encephalitis was described to me (and my family) in this way in order to make a complex condition more understandable. The thing with Encephalitis, like many other medical conditions, is that variations are possible and just as every situation and variation of the illness may be different, so might the words which are used to describe them. I can only share from my own experience in this respect.

9. Relatively Speaking

I'm weary of April. Ever since the GP put back feeling better to the end of the year, April has felt longer as if it too, like my recovery, has decided to drag itself out. I'm being mindful of the "rest, rest, rest" instruction but, for all the reasons I'm now completely bored and fed up with, it seems impossible to do this effectively.

Instead, I continue my quest to get back to normal by adding in a little thing here, an extra activity there, to get me back on my feet in a more productive way. My latest additional activities focus on two things: going out and being at home - *my* home.

I have friends, Gordon and Carol, who I met when I first moved down to Hastings; a husband and wife team who renovated the house I'd bought in readiness for my move. We bonded together as my home took shape and they've remained in contact as friends. Actually they've been incredibly helpful over this whole illness and my in-limbo situation, checking on the house for me and taking care of odd jobs. They are on my regular call-list (I still take every opportunity to talk to my friends, however one-sided the conversations) and so I call them with a special request. I experience something close to delight, a long-forgotten sensation which feels like a shiver, when they agree that next time they plan to go to the house, they will pick me up, so that I can come home with them for a while.

My list-making takes on new vigour, during these intervening days whilst I wait for the visit to come around. All my 'spare' time weighs heavily upon me. OK, so I know that it's resting and recovery time, I've been told that often enough, but I can't shake the sense that I should be doing something and, of course, sleep and relaxation don't tend to come hand-in-hand for me, so rest times become list times as I plan my to-dos for my visit home.

It's a strange sensation, writing a to-do list of things which I anticipate may need doing, either by Carol, Gordon or even myself. It's hard to remember what's involved, what the nuances and routines of my home are, partly because my memory has been so erased but also partly, I suppose, because the very act of returning there won't in itself be an act of returning to my old routine. Far from it, in fact.

#

Nevertheless, the day comes around and I'm full of anticipation as I sit in the car, being taken home. Home. To my own front door. To my own garden, which I'm eager to see. Although April's done its best to depress me, I love this time of year and I can't wait to see the spring bloom of my garden. Despite it's tiny size, my careful planting over the years means that my little patch offers its own colourful show throughout most of the spring and summer. I picture it, or at least what I think I remember of it. As we drive, I'm entranced by the soft sunlight which dances on my lap, knowing that the same rays will also be playing with the flowers, whilst the breeze encourages their dance. In my mind, I can see them nod in acknowledgement of my return and secretly, as much as today's about being at home, I actually hope to join Gordon for at least a short while, in tending to the garden. Truly, as we drive along, I cannot wait.

This part of the visit indeed fulfils all of my expectations. As Gordon parks the car in a serendipitous space on the street right outside my own home, I'm greeted by the cheery waves of the lilies blooming and bouncing in my front garden. Despite the fact that I'd forgotten their presence and that this part of April would offer them in their full glory, it feels like a fitting welcome back. Whilst Gordon unlocks the door I lurk on the path, unsteady on my sticks, gazing in wonderment at the scent and splendour of my lilies.

Eventually, I tear myself away, eager to step into the familiarity of home, deciding as I do so that once I've set Carol and Gordon up with their jobs, I'll then bask in the haven of home and maybe complete a few of those jobs on my list myself. I don't get far into the hall though, before my delusions of familiarity, much less productivity, fall away like mud on the doormat.

I don't know this hall at all. I look around it in wonderment, with the detached appraisal of a prospective buyer, as if I am a stranger viewing my own home. The boots in the hall, the nick-nacks here and there, even the family photographs on the walls are as unfamiliar to me as the length, breadth and decoration of the hall itself.

I steady myself on my sticks and follow Carol into the living room where, once again, portraits of strangers smile down on me. At least one of these strangers is the smiling woman I know was me. I don't know if I want to laugh or cry. Be careful what you wish for, springs to mind, like the thief's last laugh. I'm home, where I wanted to be, but I don't belong here. Gordon is chatting brightly about the chores to be done in the back garden but between my reduced hearing and the loud pounding in my chest, I really can't hear what he's saying. My heart is like a cartoon, beating with an exaggerated volume and colour outside of my body, but with panic, not passion or happiness. Somehow, between his chat and my aimless nodding of assent, Gordon's list of garden chores is established.

As he sets off to work, I turn away from the watchful gaze of the expectant, strangers on the wall, mortified by their presence. Unsteady as ever, but slightly more so as I seem to be trembling, I turn to Carol. She's getting ready to run the hoover through for me and I don't really want to sit whilst she hoovers round me; the ease of her actions reminds me of how reduced my own abilities are and her functional movement in the room will only encourage the flickers and movements I see from the corners of my eyes. There's not a lot else I can do, but I need to be doing something, so I do what I am best at: I shuffle about my own living room which feels as alien as a hotel foyer, moving bits of paper from one place to another. I open the post and sort it into piles: rubbish or items to take back to Sam's to deal with.

When this becomes too much, within a shockingly short time actually, I return to the front step to regard my lilies, until it's time to lock up the house again. The house. Where my word choice often fails me, my selection of that word is deliberate and truthful: as we drive away I realise that on the journey here, I was coming home but now, on the way back, it's become 'the house', it feels no more my home than Sam's does.

#

As April ticks towards May, my days start to take on a more notable pattern and routine and slowly, within this, I seem to be making what others measure as progress. I'm still not able to go out alone, but I have friends from my choir who drop by and pick me up, to take me for coffee in town or at one of their homes.

Now, I know this sounds like I'm also starting to enjoy something dangerously like a social life, but the reality is that it's not really so sociable or enjoyable. Sure, I have some lovely friends who mean very well, but gatherings in a group, even a small one, leave me just as I was when my brothers visited: on the outside, looking in. On the phone, I'm not impeded by the social propriety of following a stream of conversation, because anyone talking to me on the phone knows I can't really hear them, so my words flow and generally, the other person listens, whereas in these cosy coffee groups I can neither hear the conversation properly nor keep up. Already lacking in confidence from being out and about whilst incontinent, my lack of hearing or ready conversation makes interactions stilted. I'm also aware that, once again, I'm trying to play the part of someone getting better, to fulfil the illusion of others' expectations, inspired by my filled-out face and fragile hope.

Just as much, I find myself impatient. God forgive me, these are my friends after all ... but are they though? Sometimes we run into other people from choir who are breathlessly enthusiastic and emphatic about the fact I'm "looking so much better" and that we too "must meet for coffee." Real friends notice the difference in me, notice that this 'better' is relatively speaking, a comparative illusion and, to be honest, with my real friends, I'm not obliged to 'perform'. So, I don't see why I should be obliged to perform in the face of the patronising sympathy of those who pass on their platitudes and then go about their own business. Of course it is their right, but it's my right not to have to perform to ease their own conscience or their need to gloss over what has happened to me. I deserve better than that.

#

Sam and I sometimes pop into town too, a bit more now, although I don't mooch like I used to. Shopping's something I used to enjoy, but at the moment it takes up too much of my energy and concentration just to move around and the sensory overload from the movement of other shoppers and the glaring lights and blaring sounds from some of the stores can be just overwhelming.

I do like to go with Sam and the baby though; it's a normal mother-daughter-granddaughter activity, so I push myself where possible to be able to do this, although there's little I want in the shops for myself. I can't buy clothes and what's more, I don't want to. It's not just the fact that it would it be too much for me to have to try them on, there's also the honest truth: I have no idea what size I am now and I don't want that experience of going for my usual size and finding myself one, two or even three sizes bigger.

The thing is, I've ballooned with these continuing steroids. I know that the full moon of my face is nothing compared to my thicker waist and rounded belly, I don't need a label in a garment to tell me the awful truth. I'll stick with the loose, predominantly elasticated wardrobe I've got until I'm better or at least until I'm off the Supersize-Me steroids, whichever comes soonest!

What's more, as most of my clothing is still at my own home, and also because my recall of things is still so abysmal, getting off the steroids and being back home will bring me the equivalent of a whole 'new' wardrobe to discover. So, at this point I save my money rather than waste it on clothes, although I'm tempted by the occasional pretty scarf, to cheer these long days and add something different to the repetitive nature of the elasticated ensembles that I do actually wear at the moment.

I also buy bits and pieces for Evie - it's lovely to buy baby clothes, which seem so much more varied than when my own children were small. I also help Sam out by keeping an eye on the pushchair whilst she goes to pay, or has to hunt through racks in inconvenient corners of shops. I don't mind doing this at all, it's proper grandmother stuff and I can do it!

#

Although my counselling job is on hold, I'm still trying to go into my business office with some kind of regularity, both to help me get back into the swing of it and to re-establish my 'self', if that makes sense. This business is what I am / was and it's essential to me to reconnect with it.

#

As the 1st of May arrives it's especially important for me to mark the dawning of a brand new month, which takes me farther away from the horrors of the thief's rampage and closer to the GP's end of the year recovery, so I've made sure of coming into the office today.

I manage to do several little tasks and a considerable amount of paper shuffling but in amongst my activities, I'm aware of an awful noise, like a grating, inefficient cappuccino machine. I speak to my colleague, who shows no sign of hearing it at all, to try and gauge what he thinks. My heart sinks to my boots. I can barely hear what he's saying. The hospital said that my hearing loss was 40% and 70% but I can't remember which ear is which and today they both seem bad ... just, so much worse, this can't be right. I feel like shaking my head to clear my ears – I just don't seem to be able to hear anything at all. Maybe it's from the perpetual swelling of my throat, the ongoing sign of my struggling immune system or perhaps I'm just a bit congested?

#

Today's a big day for me: lunch with old business colleagues from London, but just like yesterday, my ears feel strange. Lorraine arrives to pick me up and take me to meet up with everyone but that same strange whizzing fills my ears and insinuates itself where I should be able to hear at least a little of the conversation. The lunch becomes an old cine film being played out around me: a silent movie where I have to concentrate on everyone's expressions to work out the action, see how everyone's feeling. I watch their lips, fascinated by the speed and variety of word watching. I am a voyeur of the conversation, not a part of it.

Sam picks me up on her way home, to return me once more to her house. I know that I should be full of animation and excitement about catching up with everyone but I don't have the strength to perform. As it turns out, a performance would be unnecessary, as Sam can see and, ironically, hear from the exasperated repetition and necessary volume of her own voice, that there seems to be a real problem with my ears at the moment.

#

She drives me the next day to the emergency doctor. As I make my way into his surgery, on my sticks, he greets me like a long-lost friend, although as far as I'm concerned he's a complete stranger to me. Through painstaking conversation and much gesticulating and repetition of fact at a volume you'd complain to your neighbours about, it turns out that he's the doctor who was called out to Sam's house; the one who admitted me to hospital on 29th January. He says that he thought I had a brain tumour when he admitted me. I'm not sure what to do with this information. I'm guessing I should thank him for everything ... from his diligence and professionalism on that night, to the fact he's remembered me from then, when I can't even remember myself or that, thankfully, he's now referring me urgently back to the Ear, Nose and Throat (ENT) consultant at the very same hospital. I think I do thank him, but I can't remember exactly why, especially as I leave his room exactly the same as I came into it – deaf, incontinent and struggling on my sticks. Thank you for saving me? *This* me? Thank you for *this*?

#

Of course, there's a wait for the appointment to come through and May marches on, right through my ears. The tension in Sam's house continues, only now it's been raised to a level that's probably commensurate with volume I need to engage with anything at all around me. Sam seems to be cross with me for this deterioration, whilst I'm cross with myself for not being better, for being ill in the first place and with the world for not understanding how trapped and isolated I feel inside this badly behaved body.

#

Despite the fact that reading is still a skill I am trying to re-learn, two of my sisters send me two books by Bernadette Bohan, both named The Choice, both of which relate the story of this lady's journey through cancer and the lifestyle choices incumbent on her during her battles. Although delighted to receive an unexpected gift, I'm completely confused by it ... I don't have cancer, what are they thinking?

It takes me some time and more than a little painstaking reading of the blurb and introductions of both books to realise that Bernadette Bohan is a woman like me ... an Irish woman, a mother, stricken suddenly by a life-changing illness. Unlike myself and my illness, a business woman with Viral Encephalitis, this lady is a much admired Irish author who had cancer twice. The second time around, she worked out her own programme of treatment to complement the better effects and minimise the worst of the medical treatment she also had to undergo. The first book is about her initial journey through breast cancer, the second about her choice of treatment and the methods she used. Although still slightly confounded by my sisters' reasoning behind sending the books, I'm sure there's a message in there for me, so I resolve to try to read them.

In truth, trapped by the increasing isolation from the deafness, which has now mostly curtailed my efforts towards those social gatherings of taking a coffee with friends, I have plenty of time to try to improve my reading so I make every attempt, whenever I can, to read the books. I'm intrigued by the author's fortitude and also by my sisters' choice of books. As my reading painfully progresses, I realise that the act of trying to read them is in fact enforcing why my sisters sent them in the first place: to share the tale of one lady's grit and determination not to be beaten. I am humbled by both Bernadette's journey and by my sisters' thoughtfulness. Although my isolation has left the time and space for my reading, these books have left me feeling less alone.

I phone my sisters to thank them. As I speak to one of them, she tells me that I am shouting down the phone to her, as if it is she who is deaf. I try to describe the irony of very noisy deafness; it's like walking against a strong wind on the beach, where the wind not only fills your ears but causes other sounds to carry on and away, not stopping to be understood or processed. So here we are: she has to shout from her end as my only chance of hearing her and I forget we're not on that windy beach of our childhood and I shout back. It reminds me of our few occasions of raised voices in those spectacularly explosive teenage years, when my father would enter the room and rail at us: "you're shouting at each other like men in a storm!" How strange then, that now this is how I feel about every verbal interaction, shouting against the storm in my own ears.

#

The books, coinciding with my now worsening hearing, are having another curious effect on me. I've always been a woman of faith yet since contracting VE, faith has fast become another side of myself which seems to have been lost to me.

Despite my ears, I decide to take the opportunity for a catch up with two of my friends from the church, Pat and Elizabeth. In the event, it turns out to be a fairly spontaneous lunch in Elizabeth's high decked garden looking out over the sea in St Leonard's. The weather is fine and after such a grey, insular start to the year, it's lovely to feel the sun on my shoulders and to gaze out at the gentle roll and swell of the sea. Over lunch, I have to explain again what Viral Encephalitis is as, with many people, including myself before it happened to me, they haven't really heard of it, much less understand the effects it has. I give a fairly stilted (and possibly loud) overview of the current effects, although my loudness interspersed with silence, arrival on wobbly legs and walking sticks, plus my handbag full of Tena Lady pads would have served equally well if a physical demonstration were required.

There's a respectful silence when I finish, or at least without the white noise of my ears there would have been. Pat regards me gently and apparently says "that will test your faith" but of course I don't hear her. Helpfully, she writes it down for me.

"I don't think I have any!" I say, simply. And I don't think I do. A direct casualty of the thief; an indirect response to my year so far perhaps, or a crisis borne of realising that, like Bernadette Bohan, I can only rely on myself to get me through the road ahead? Who knows?

For their part, Pat and Elizabeth are surprisingly understanding and unsurprisingly forgiving of my lapse into a frank response. I share with them that I recognise the problem and that I have contacted the local branch of The White Eagle Group, a UK-wide spiritual, healing group. Pat's response is as quick as it is pragmatic.

"What for?" she asks. "When you can join a healing group right here in your own church? There's a charismatic group now, it's every Tuesday 8-9 and the healer is the parish priest." By the end of the lunch, we have arranged to meet there and then, the following Tuesday.

#

So, it's the appointed hour to join the charismatic group and off I go, deaf as a post by this time, to find Pat waiting outside, waving me in. I make my way into the sanctuary of the church ante-room she directs me to, craving both comfort and familiarity from the atmosphere and fabric of the building, but finding little of either. In truth, it's not my regular church but I am vaguely familiar with it from when I first moved to St. Leonard's, I came here a few times as Sam and Simon were married here.

There are readings, which I cannot hear and there is singing. Of course, I realise, there would be singing. I feel that I recognise some of the parishioners and I watch their mouths in wonder and with increasing anxiety. The only thing I recognise is *Hills and Mountains Praise the Lord*. I watch the call outs and the responses, trying to match the movement of their mouths, but finding myself instead farcically out of sync, tears running down my face, trying to keep up with the hands raised in Hallelujahs.

When at last this church-based purgatory is over, Pat comes to find me, accompanied by a woman I don't really recognise.

"Tell this lady what you had," Pat suggests and, as I launch into my now-familiar yet testing and probably over-loud explanation of my degenerated state, one of the passing "hallelujah" women appears to overhear.

"Was that you?" she interrupts, before continuing. "I felt so much healing. You must come for the next healing in two weeks."

I mumble a non-committal response although slightly humbled by her absolute faith in the idea of achieving a level of healing which just continues to elude me. My son-in-law pulls up to pick me up and sees us saying our goodbyes. As we drive home, he reminds me that he and Sam had spoken about a lady from the church who was part of Evie's christening prep day, a lady who embodied such absolute, infallible faith that he was amazed. Sure enough, it was this lady he'd just seen me saying goodbye to. Clearly her faith isn't in question then, but mine certainly is. I resolve to think about all of this, during those hideous waking hours of the darkness. But then, once those interminable hours and their ghouls come around again, that resolve is soon lost to me.

#

Tomorrow comes of course, although it's today by now. I spend it with Carol and Gordon, at the house which is supposed to be my home. I am doing too much - the doctors' mantra of "rest" is still just an offensive four-lettered word to me, in my desperate attempts to find something to trigger my association with these bricks and mortar, these decorations and photographs, items pretty or purposeful which made up my life up until 28th January. I pull belongings out from here and there, before Gordon locks up my house and drops me back to Sam's house – neither of which is my home - with a box to check through, to sort out, to identify myself by.

I return dog-tired to my room after dinner, laying on the bed to recover my legs a little from the climb up the stairs. My eye catches the box, including a box of Avalon cards from Louise Hay collection, dumped where I'd left them. Don't ask me why, but my sister had given me them for Christmas a long while back and I had been listening to the Louise Hay tapes at the end of 2007 on 'you can heal yourself'. As I handle the cards, I'm surprised to find that this memory's there, as if amongst the cards itself: I'm establishing an association between myself, some of my belongings and my memories. I should feel energised or excited by this, I think to myself and I pick out cards absent-mindedly as I wait for my emotions to catch up with my thoughts and my actions. They don't. Instead I find I have picked up the cards 33.5.6, all of which pose the question: what is my purpose? I think this is the point where my faith should answer, should be shouting itself as loud as the men in the storm, or the hallelujah of the lady of great faith from the church. But there is just the storm, not the shouting, certainly no answer driven by blind, humble faith. I can't answer the question and, as we're being honest, it's a question which still haunts me ... it's one which I think has never been answered.

#

To be honest, where having faith in being able to hear again is concerned, I set more store by the ENT appointment and spend my days alternately eagerly waiting for it to arrive yet trying to convince myself not to expect too much. I'm reminded of my bargaining with God whilst in hospital. One day I say to Sam, "if this (my hearing) is all I have to deal with, I will be OK." I think I'm resigning myself to there being some issue, some silence to come. What I don't bargain for is the dreaded Tinnitus which now more regularly replaces all normal sounds.

I have so much to ask about this and my many other issues so of course I continue to busy myself with my question lists for this ENT appointment and the many other appointments which are starting to come through. It's like having my bulging business diary back again except, instead of booking in appointments to extend, expand and enjoy my life – everything my work diary had represented - I'm now booking in appointments to try to recover aspects of me, of that life or, in the spirit of being positive, trying to minimise the impact of this new me.

When I finally attend the ENT appointment, I'm pleased and horrified in equal measures to be offered hearing aids. Along with the walking sticks and incontinence pads, I'm starting to feel like one of those models in the strange 'helpful' appliance brochures which come with other catalogues and magazines. The only difference is that those models are smiling about it. Still, if it means I can hear, enjoy conversations, tune back into my beloved music, really then the hearing aids would be a blessing ... wouldn't they?

At first, snugly fitted, it seems that this will be the case ... these will be appliances which will help rather than exaggerate my needs, they will amplify aspects of myself I've been looking for since the thief struck. I wait, as patiently as I possibly can, whilst the audiologist fiddles with the fitting and the batteries and then, finally, these miracles of modern science are switched on. Instantly, a rage of white noise fills my head with a dazzling kaleidoscope of confusion. The audiologist is apologetic but that can't change the facts: my condition is such that, apparently, the aids serve only to amplify the tinnitus.

#

Sam remains a stalwart as my "fortnight's recovery" continues into its second month since leaving hospital. Although I can't seem to get us over this impasse of pain that my illness has caused, one thing has changed - for me at least. Since finding a loose strand of myself in the box of cards from my sister and bolstered by my reading of the Bohan books, I have substituted my misplaced faith in my

God for a growing faith in myself ... whoever I was, or am currently.

#

I take more visits to my house and I'm starting to want to spend more time there. I still don't know the benign, smiling faces on the wall, but they and many other things in the house are starting to become familiar. This is probably because I'm now visiting more often and more productively, but I'm starting to think that I'm feeling a sense of home-comfort from being there too.

This sense is particularly heightened when the man I have so long struggled to recognise as my son, Simon, and his wife Julie come for the weekend. They have been over several times over this period of recovery and, thankfully he's becoming much more familiar to me although when I am anxious I do fear that this is because he's been attentive and has become known to me since I've been ill, rather than becoming remembered from our whole lifetime together, that lifetime before VE.

I prepare for the visit with something as close to vigour as two walking sticks, the cloud of white noise in my head and the thick wedge of incontinence pads allow! Carol and Gordon take me to my house most days and they do the main jobs, preparing the garden and the house whilst I play house and practise preparing meals for my family. When the house is ready, Carol and Gordon take me shopping. To my absolute delight, during Simon and Julie's stay, I am able to have both of my children, their spouses and my beautiful "baby girl" to my house for dinner. I have a sense of normal, just like when I'm standing by Evie's pushchair whilst Sam mooches or queues up. This is something I can do, this is what a mother does.

#

Although I'm still very caught up in my dependence on others, I do end the month on a high note where my independence is concerned - I make my first outing alone. I've managed to find a well reputed local acupuncturist who, fortuitously, lives in the next road. Sam's booked the appointment for me and she drops me off. Of course I'd rather be seeing Dr. Shen in Sutton, but I just can't get there at the moment, so this will have to do.

It's a horribly long appointment, two hours because of being a new patient. We spend the first hour going through my history, which is grim for all concerned and, once more, I start crying and can't seem to stop. A shock seems to take hold of me when I have to talk about this, this whole experience, the person I was and now am.

The second hour is the acupuncture treatment. It's a very different approach to what I'm used to, but it's here and I can get to it. I guess it's also good to have a safe outlet for the crying, because this basically has been another crying session.

I don't feel too terrible when I come out, just extremely tired of course. After being inside and being so upset, the warm May afternoon feels fresh on my face and I recall how comforting, how freeing it is to just take a walk in the fresh air. So, I make the decision, then and there, to walk back. It took us five minutes to drive here and I estimate that it'll probably take me about forty five minutes to get back. Although I'm feeling weak and of course I'm reliant on my sticks, I set out, with as determined a step as I can muster. And I'm doing it .... I'm out and about, one foot kind of in front of the other, purposefully and independently walking back to Sam's!

And the time? The first thing I do as I walk into the kitchen is look at the clock. I'm amazed to see that it's taken me just fifteen minutes ... yet it had seemed so far, like I was walking so far. I guess though, where my confidence and independence are concerned, I have indeed made great strides today.

10. Cry Baby

June is proving to be a strange month. I visit my home yet cannot be there full-time as my capabilities are still too limited and my hearing makes it extremely hard to be independent. My medical appointments are starting to come through thick and fast and I drag myself along to each one. Of course I go complete with a list and a continued hope that something useful will be offered, something which will remedy the situation I still find myself in. No such luck, yet.

I'm still regularly obliged to visit the GP along with my on-going symptoms, including my hearing, palpitations and bizarrely sore legs, each seeming to exist in their own independent hot, then cold and painful state, from the rest of my body. "It's the medication," the GP announces. "Contact your neurologist and tell him you need therapy."

Of course, I can't manage that kind of phone conversation now, so my son-in-law Simon calls for me. The secretary, professional and perfunctory, tells us that she will look into it.

Meanwhile, my isolation has stepped up a notch as, conversely, although I am slightly more able in myself to be picked up by friends for a coffee or a trip into town, my hearing and the trials and errors with hearing aids make it impossible to interact sensibly and even coherently with others. Sure, I have my own side of the conversation but even that is becoming tiresome, to myself as well as others.

So, when I'm not visiting my house or attending medical appointments, I spend a considerable amount of time trying to kid myself I'm still usefully hands-on (although ears off) in running my company. Being at work is a great escape but in truth, just getting there is enough for me - doing it is another story. Practical difficulties aside, there is also the conflict within myself that comes because I need to reimburse – or acknowledge - other people's efforts. However, when I try to, the gesture is dismissed and I feel rejected and altogether far less worthwhile. As a therapist I know I should approach this by just accepting these efforts of others as kindly gestures, in the spirit of a gift. The problem is that those offering the efforts also offer up the fact that they are so very busy and tied up in other ways, so it feels like I have imposed on them twice, with both my need and my gratitude, without even trying.

So it goes without saying that I am mostly still at Sam's house. Three months after my predicted fortnight of residence, I'm still here and the toll is showing on all of us. For my part, I know the current daily dosage of steroids continue to reduce my capacity for sleep (restful or otherwise) and give me a strange fervour and impatience which borders on urgency over the tiniest things. In the face of my hideously slow progress, prolonged imposition on my family and this medically induced-impatience, I feel I receive little patience in return: the ultimate irony of still being very much a patient myself.

#

Thankfully there are other events to serve as a distraction. Sam and Simon have been attending their christening class at the church because of course Evie's christening is coming up at the end of the month. I watch them making their plans and arrangements and try to assist, but I feel no more involved than I did in that rugby match two months ago.

It also troubles me that I have no christening gown to hand down, from mother to daughter so, instead I offer to pay for one. My suggestion is welcomed gratefully and Sam suggests we take a trip to town together to choose one. Despite the auditory harassment and sensory overload of the town centre, I'm pleased to be here as a real part of the search, of the event. Together we find the ideal robe, beautifully intricate and very pretty, yet also traditional – important to Sam and, in the context of our church, extremely appropriate. The unfamiliar sensation of joy rises in me as Sam and I seem, at last, to be in complete accord about something and I also feel blissfully content that I have fulfilled a vital grandmotherly role.

But, it's not as easy as that. I watch the baby's pushchair whilst Sam goes to the counter and I wait eagerly in the wings to pay. However, Sam returns without the garment, resolute that it will be held behind the counter for her so that Simon can come down and join her in that final decision. I'm guessing that my old self would have understood this completely, it's a family decision after all. Unfortunately, my pharmaceutically-enhanced paranoia bursts my small bubble of contentment with a spiteful, internal tirade of resentment, railing at me that my input was just not good enough and was probably, like my continued presence around the house, at best just tolerated.

#

My sister Frances is coming over soon, which also breaks things up a bit and gives me a genuine reason, other than the desperate need to hang on to every passing thought I have, to make another list. My handwriting's come a long way, although it's still something of a scribble, but rather than let it disgust me I now regard it as compromise I have to put up with: I don't want to be the author of such scrawl but I do want access to those thoughts and ideas which will otherwise slip away unless I take every opportunity to commit them as written words. So, a to-do list for when Frances comes is, well, top of my to-do list! It's not much to look at:

1) Order baby gift.
2) Things to get: dress for christening; baby bible.
3) Go to bank.

A fairly innocuous list but one behind which lays a hidden agenda and still a hidden sadness: I must do these whilst Frances is here, whilst I have the additional support that I need.

#

Also on the calendar, towards the beginning of the month, is my first Hydrotherapy session. The Neurology department's physiotherapist told me quite clearly "you are entitled to sessions" and I can remember saying to her "I am entitled to get well."

I'm starting to wonder now if this road of referrals and on-going department shuffles is what that kind Encephalitis Society man meant all that time ago when, despite my assured "I'll be better soon" he advised that I must get referred back to the neurology department. More than anyone else, professional or family, I'm starting to trust the Encephalitis Society's guidance the most.

So, I've been looking forward to this intervention, but that's before I realise just how much hassle is involved in this hour's therapy. Of course, I've been on the waiting list for a while now and it seems to me that the whole system has an ironic undercurrent of waiting – and then waiting some more.

Firstly, I have spent an incredible amount of time on the waiting list to actually access my six sessions of therapy, my "entitlement". Then, although the therapy is sixty minutes long, it turns out I have to allow four and a half hours out of my whole day for it, all because of my damn hearing. I have hospital transport, you see, for which I've to be ready two hours before the session time, as part of the general pick-up slot, within which they'll arrive at some point to collect me. The trouble is, I can't rely on being able to hear them pull up outside or knock on the door when they arrive for me. And if I miss them? I'll not only lose my therapy session, but also my access to the therapy as a whole, according to the hospital rules.

My enthusiasm for finally accessing the hydrotherapy ironically sinks like a stone as I prepare for my debut session by lurking in a panicked, paranoid state at the window, afraid to leave it for a moment. I off-set some of my panic by making sure I've got the key in my hand because I'm worried I'll forget to bring it when I have to leave the house in that "they're here!" flurry. The idea of being locked out terrifies me, so here I stand, clutching the key, frightened to move just in case I miss the arrival of the transport and wondering what awaits me at the hospital.

In the event, compared to the discomfort of the wait: the sitting, standing and leaning of my aching body, the key panic, along with the conflict of the incontinence and not being able to dash from the window to the loo and back again, the hydrotherapy itself is quite a doddle. At least there's no sinking on my part there: the steroid air bag of my body seems to float pretty well!

#

I still hanker for my natural remedies of course and now that I've proved myself vaguely independent enough to walk to the most local (to Sam's) acupuncture clinic, I do so as often as I am able to which is usually dependent on two things: physically, whether I'm up for it, as my days still generally alternate between pretty bad and less bad – I'm hoping for what I'd call a "good day" any time soon; and financially, as none of the alternative treatments are cheap and I'm still waiting to find out where I stand with my health insurance after all this illness and yes, after all this time too! The waiting lists and limited sessions of NHS treatments and rehabilitations make privately funded options seem extremely appealing, but of course the wait with them is for the insurance company to decide whether my VE is covered or not. Either way, it's more waiting, more recovery time spent in hiatus.

#

Speaking of waiting, my manager from the counselling service has come to see me today. He's been so good about keeping me in touch and, in complete contrast to my own impatience at my slow progress with recovery, being so brittle and cross about it that I could just snap at any moment, he just seems so patient, so accepting.

As usual I take him at his professional best and launch into my own update of the medical circles around which my life now revolves; the limited progress that I'm unable to recognise for the progress it is because to me it isn't enough; the waking nightmares; the ridiculousness of hearing aids which amplify all intrusive sound and offer little viable assistance, oh and my continued fear and anxiety that I will never be back to my old self.

Eventually, the conversation comes to the counselling service itself. Dave updates me on the recent Annual General Meeting and tells me all about who is now doing what and why. It's natural then, in this context, that we come around to talking about my position there. Obviously I'm now into my fifth month of absence, so he tells me that he has had to speak with the Trustees about needing help. His response, he relays to me, is that he could take on a temp to cover my position as a project worker. The trouble is, even as he tells me this, we both know that this isn't feasible. My role was a new post when I was appointed – it needs the continuity and development of a permanent worker.

The real solution is far more obvious and of course, in my candour I can't really think it through for all of its implications before sharing my thoughts with him. I find myself telling him that getting a temp in just won't work. Instead, I suggest that I should resign and make way for someone new to be appointed. As the words pass into the air between us, I realise that I've just relieved him of a difficult, burdensome situation, and for that I'm glad, because the situation must be intolerable for the service, yet as my manager he's always been so kind.

For my part though, there's little relief in the decision. OK, so it's one less thing to worry about, one less reason to ignore the doctors' "rest, rest, rest" and be relentlessly pushing myself instead to be well enough to fulfil all my obligations, including work. Yes, to that extent I'm relieved of a responsibility. But as he graciously accepts my suggestion, I realise that I've just added to my own emotional burdens: the whole conversation, this whole time-line of my illness and so-called progress to date has made me realise how little I am capable of. It's more than that though. Just as my hearing has put paid to my ideas about continuing as a member of the choir's community, I have just removed myself from a role in another community that I enjoyed being a part of, and one which was very much part of my future plans.

In all, I can tell he's relieved that he came yet I am relieved when he leaves. As I close the door behind him, the unheard, conclusive snap of the latch feels like yet another metaphor for my whole life since my illness began.

#

Frances arrives and is more than happy to spend time with me, despite my heavy dependence and to-do list, which has grown more extensive as my enthusiasm for her visit has built up. Of everyone around me, Frances has the best understanding of my hearing issues and the effect it's having on me, as she's a visiting teacher for deaf children in Ireland. She has an excellent knowledge of all sides of the issue: the medical, the routines of auditory referrals, assessments and treatment options, and of course speaks the relevant language of acronyms and denotations.

One day, during her visit, I have an appointment at the audiology clinic in nearby Bexhill, so Frances accompanies me as both my sister and my advocate. Having lost so many of my own accomplishments to the thief, I appreciate hers and, although I can't hear what she's saying to the audiologist, I'm pleased and grateful for her knowledge and her fortitude on my behalf. Somehow, my world is less noisily silent when she's around and when she has to go back home, the weight of isolation once again presses in on me, despite the fact that I now have two new hearing aids to reattach me to the rest of the world.

#

Why do I continue to wake up crying at the same time as the baby? I waken with tears on my cheeks, not knowing why this little baby seems to be a catalyst for everything I feel about being locked inside my own body. It's hard to describe the hurt I feel as I acknowledge the things I cannot do with her. Although her mother says I do lots with her, to me it doesn't come from the right place. There's none of that easy maternal spontaneity of scooping up, crouching down and cuddling – it's all too much of an effort which takes time to rally my body for. I just want to be able to pick her up and to take little walks with her on her toddling feet, to do this would be such a joy but I need to think about everything, my sticks, the stairs, the garden. When I think of what I could be doing with her, the kind of grandma role I could have, I experience a physical pain in my chest which I think may be my heart, literally, breaking.

As painful too is the situation where I'm not allowed to express this hurt, explain how I feel. It's hard to get anyone to believe how scared and anxious I am and how self-destructive this feeling is. Six months on, I'm constantly being told "you're doing well", yet deep down in myself I know there is so much more to do, to regain, to be able to show, in order to begin to be anywhere near the person I'd recognise as myself, my old self.

Yes, my energy is coming back, there is no doubt, but I feel so tired at the same time. The emotional feelings are so strong that when I talk about any of this, I just find my carefully steered ship of the self crashing against the rocks, once more wrecked. This wretchedness is so easily, conveniently dismissed as being a result of the condition or a result of the medication, because I guess that's a more palatable truth, an easier understanding than to acknowledge that actually, this is how I genuinely feel.

#

I remain enthusiastic about the christening though. Living so far from my own Irish-rooted family, I've always loved get-togethers and my son has confirmed that he'll be coming. I'm so looking forward to seeing him and spending time with him.

Out of the blue, my brother telephones to say that he and his daughter have booked to come and see me, co-incidentally on the same weekend as the christening. I'm starting to put serious thought into whether I should try to stay at my own house with them, as they've not seen my house, when my son Simon announces that his wife's got the time off too, so she'll be joining him for the weekend. This helps to decide things for me: I want to have them all to stay with me, in my own home. It will make things easier for Sam and it will mean that I can at least pretend to be my old self, in my own home (sticks, aids, pads and hallucinations aside, of course).

#

So my days take on a new shape of house-preparations at both ends: Sam's house for her visitors and likewise my house, my home, for mine. The trouble is, the whole new shape of my steroid-bound personality seems to be impacting significantly: I have a growing sense of impatience and urgency which is almost a teeth grinding paranoia. I simply cannot tolerate this waiting game as the minutes, hours and days tick by until I get to see the rest of my family. I can barely contain myself: I'm like a child marking off the dates till Christmas, but with less of a child-like charm and more of a stroppy adolescent frustration!

And in amongst all of these preparations I have, what is to me, a very exciting opportunity. Sam's been invited to a reunion in a school in London where she worked several years ago. She's keen to go but Simon's going to be away that weekend, so I've offered to go with her for the company and it seems that, like me, she thinks that would be a good idea.

As there are plenty of activities for her to be getting on with up there, as part of the reunion, I suggest to her that perhaps I could take the opportunity to go and see my herbalist. After the "I don't buy into that" response last time I broached the subject, I feel a little nervous about it, but as it turns out Sam agrees that it could fit in well if the appointment's around 4 pm. The fact that we are then able to book it in, on the very day, at the given time seems to me to be entirely serendipitous. Once again I'm in the happy, although exhausting situation of having something else to be obsessively and excitedly anxious about!

It turns out to be a day of surprising outcomes, but not necessarily in the ways I might have predicted. Dr. Shen is delighted to see me and is full of advice and recommendations for the best way to manage my recovery. Our previous communication difficulties are even more exacerbated by my deafness but we not only manage to communicate, we even have a little laugh over it. She prescribes the usual concoction of herbs for me to have for two weeks and a month's worth of sachets of anti-infection tea to be taken twice a day.

I also have my acupuncture from her – who would have thought that you could long so for someone to stick their needles in you, and to be so grateful for it? But here I am, so very grateful. Being here feels like old times, which is healing in itself and on top of this I have every faith that what she is doing for me will help me to recover. There's a real sense of coming home, being here with her again. I walk out feeling different, which is not a surprise because I knew I would, this is why I have been yearning to get back here. I wish I'd had the strength and the ability to get here sooner.

#

"You seem stronger today," Sam comments to me the next day, with a smile. She's right of course, after my acupuncture yesterday I *am* stronger.

"I knew I would be, if only I could go to her," I reply, another of my broad statements of absolute truth.

"Well, there's no reason why you can't," Sam suggests.

I'm a bit concerned that there's an undercurrent here, something I'm missing, and I really don't want to say the wrong thing, what with the good day we had yesterday and the christening coming up. I remind her, in the gentlest way I possibly can, which I'm painfully aware still has all the grace of a blunderbuss, of the reasons why I haven't been – lack of opportunity, lack of support to do so, lack of faith in my own understanding of what is good for my body, for my soul.

To my surprise, instead of reacting to this, Sam acknowledges it for what it is. She admits her own fears of the whole situation surrounding my illness, revealing that her faith had to remain in the medical, pharmaceutical route to my recovery. It seems that, like me, she had neither energy nor faith enough to expend on other things, the acupuncture being one of these "other things", indeed she'd said at the time "I don't buy into that at all" and of course at the time I was too ill to force the issue or find someone else to take me, so I didn't go.

Sam admits that at the time she really couldn't see the wood for the trees and with this admission a spontaneous warmth of true understanding passes between us. This feels like another example of our confused cause and effect over whose issue is whose and how lack of clarity and openness can bring confusion. I know Sam has learned a valuable lesson here and for my part, I too come away from this weekend wiser and, I think, a little more hopeful.

#

Of course the appointments continue amongst the planning. It's another Thursday, another hydro day. As usual, I'm at the window, waiting for the transport. The phone rings and I am wracked with anguish: to answer it is to move away from the window; to move away from the window puts me in a panic that I may miss the transport; but the call might be important, and I might miss that too.

I answer the call, breathless from having to move somewhat swiftly and from panic. The call itself is of course prolonged by the woman at the other end trying to make herself heard as well as understood. Somehow I do grasp what she's trying to say: the session is cancelled, a mix up over numbers leaves me being the last to be told. Even as I replace the phone I find myself drawn back to my spot at the window to ponder this change of plan. So now what do I do? I could go to my house for a while but no, that is arranged for tomorrow. I start to dither over what to do now, I can't decide: stay or go to my house? Call a taxi to get there? Or not? Just stay put?

I didn't used to be like this. The old me would have shrugged pragmatically and decided on an alternative activity, or at least have put the kettle on for a cuppa whilst pondering my options. Instead, this me can't manage the information, it feels like something inside has imploded; I cannot cope with the change. What was arranged was set, I've built my day around it and I just cannot see how to adjust to the alteration of plans, it just does not factor into my thinking; I'm supposed to be standing by the window, waiting for my transport. In the absence of a sensible alternative, I stay at the window, staring blankly at the world outside, hoping it will help me decide what to do.

#

It's now the middle of the month, almost three months to the day since I was discharged for my "fortnight's" recovery. Although I have the usual raging storm in my ears, I'm managing to pace myself well and I'm having a pretty good day in all. I think it's helped that I haven't gone into the office. It's amazing how something so normal, so routine for so many people, including the old me, can make such a difference to whether I can now get through my day in any reasonable kind of way. Not going into the office has given me a little better balance to my routine and my emotions.

Despite this, I've been pretty busy by relative standards: I've typed, the pace of which itself is improving slightly; written some emails; hobbled to the shop around the corner; pottered in the garden. A friend stops by for coffee and, although our conversation is fragmented with gesticulation and misunderstanding, there's a relative sense of normality to it. I've now just done some juicing and prepared tea for us all whilst Sam and Simon bath the baby.

Sam's hugged me today too, a hug like she used to, apropos nothing other than affection and enjoying a moment. She told me that I'm welcome here even if I'm feeling 100% well, which was so good to hear, so in all my day has been paced, productive and pleasant. There. A positive.

#

Then evening comes, bringing with it the night and as I lie here, wakeful and in pain, everything I have done, achieved, felt today becomes nothing. I feel empty, my mind wanders to a distant place between my head and my heart, a place of fear. Once again I find myself crying, the endless crying. I'm in my room, imprisoned by my emotions and the tears which seem to come from nowhere but are everywhere. I'm thinking things that I have never thought before and would not have believed I was capable of. As much as I feel empty, I feel cross. For every ounce of nothingness I'm also filled with a pound of darkest poison. The root of something is growing within me, as unwelcome and prolific as Japanese Knotweed. I don't know if it's anger or jealousy, but it's certainly a fear of being left out. Or is that of being left behind? Or of being forgotten?

I am shocked at my discoveries of jealousy and anger. I have never felt jealous of anybody and I know, *I know*, how destructive it can be, both from personal experience and counselling practise. I don't express anger, because to me that's the dangerous flip-side of the jealousy coin, I learned this to my cost in my married days. Of course, that doesn't mean that I never felt angry, it was just that I was a master at managing and disguising it. I always took my anger out on the house, it would be spotless, polished and vacuumed in a couple of hours and I would feel better – the equivalent for others of going for a run or to the gym.

I just need to cry, to let it all out, but I am so afraid of not getting better and so afraid that Sam doesn't really want me here, even though I know she has said the very opposite today, shouted it above the storm in my ears. I can't rationalise what I know from what I feel, what I fear. I can't believe I'm knotted with this feeling, this bitter, resentful anger. I truly believed I'd dealt with this subject over and over both in personal counselling and over four years of counselling training but all the time it's been here, screaming to be released and now it is, with tears and terrors I just can't stop! Tears and terrors that won't let me do anything other than lie awake and offer up my usual, unheard prayer.

11. New Beginnings

Just before her christening comes Evie's first celebration: her very first birthday. Of course she knows no differently bless her, she is just happy to be made a fuss of and to be fed as she would any morning. Her mum is at work today and her dad is at home with her and myself as we excitedly plan for the gifts and cards to be opened this afternoon.

I go to my acupuncture appointment at 11.30 and when I get back dad and babe are ready to go out. They offer to give me a lift to my house as I've planned to go in with flowers and bits that I have bought to cheer the place up before my visitors come for the christening on Saturday. Of course I jump at the chance (well, as much as my sticks and the effect of gravity on the incontinence allow) and spend a happy couple of hours in my house which, since I have been spending more time there and particularly since I have been preparing for family visitors, has started (despite the strangers on the wall who know different) to feel a little like home, my home.

Being at the house is good for me, I decide, especially on a day like today. I get a glimpse of the joy of this time of year when I can forget, just momentarily about my illness. The peony roses are glorious as are the lilies, all yellow and wonderful and carnations of my front garden, which still wave their excited greeting as I arrive. I stare at them for the longest time before I drag myself off to complete my chores. My enjoyment of the flowers is almost as fleeting as their own blooms, you see: it lasts for the duration of my seeing it, as I can't hold anything like this in my mind now. Although this means that I won't be able to think back and picture my flowers in my mind when I'm back at Sam's, it does mean that when I come out of my house to go back to hers, I am taken aback by their beauty, once again. With my goldfish brain there's never a same-old element to my flowers, just refreshed charm every single time.

#

It's now Thursday and the christening's all set for the weekend. Both pairs of visitors, my brother and niece, my son and daughter-in-law are due to arrive today. However, on this very day that I've been so eagerly waiting for, my enthusiasm is completely frustrated by the fact that Thursdays are still dominated by hydrotherapy. So, once again I spend over an hour before the designated session time rooted beside the front window. Not a situation I enjoy at the best of times, thanks to my bodily discomforts but today my nerves too are jangling and niggling away somewhere at the base of my neck as I angst about being caught up in the routes of the driver and routines of the hospital, potentially ending up unable to get home before everyone's due to arrive.

Now I know that to the highly flexible, professional woman I was before, this should all be of negligible consequence. But it isn't to me, this me, now. In fact, it's the source of an incomparable stress that I can feel hanging over me like a cloud, like one of those silly emoticon things with an expression of doom and steam rising from where its ears should be.

I'm cursing the driver before he even arrives (in the event early) because of the fact my ears have me scared to move, not out of ear-shot of course but out of sight of the bus. When he finally pulls up, another chirpy chappy, I'm curt with him and have no time to pretend to want banter, even if I could hear it. I just want him to put his foot down and get the deed done and, although I'm reasonably relaxed in the hydrotherapy session itself, I know I'm not getting the most from it largely because I just want to get through it and get home again. Of course, that too is also easier said than done, as I'm growlingly frustrated by the ridiculously difficult process of getting dried and getting dressed again, along with seeing to my interminable, intimate incontinence. Then there's the final wait for the availability and punctuality of the hospital transport on the return journey, of course!

I've arrived home just on 4.30 pm. My frustrations and angst have abated somewhat, partly I think because I'm safely back and haven't missed anything and partly because I'm now exhausted from the energy-sap which comes with hydrotherapy days. I think I'll do my juicing, so that I can keep up to date with my routines but also to keep my hands and mind as occupied as possible for this final stage of the waiting game, before I morph into someone even more unbearable, not the person I want to be to greet my family with at all!

#

It's Friday morning and I've wakened as if drugged. OK, of course I am significantly medicated, but today it feels more like that hangover feeling from late nights and fast living, but I know that fast-living's not responsible; it is indeed the late night. Last night, after Simon and Julie arrived first at Sam's house we had a lovely dinner, just like the one at my house last month: my children, their spouses and the baby. Although of course I couldn't hear too much, it was great to bask in the delights of their company, of seeing my children both together. As the dinner progressed, a quiet joy and calm slowly seemed to replace that reckless impatience of the past few weeks, and particularly melting my anxieties of the day itself, with gradual, poultice-like warmth.

At the end of the meal, we'd decamped to my house to wait for my brother and niece who, unfortunately hadn't arrived until around 11 pm, which for me felt extremely late into the night. Of course we'd prolonged the moment because my brother Joe has never seen my house before and there seemed to be lots of catching up to do even before we all finally fell into bed – almost literally in my case! It's strange, for all that my relationship with sleep is very poor, there must be some truth in the each of my many doctors' advocating "rest, rest, rest" because it was clear last night, with my enhanced slurred speech, word loss and even poorer balance, coupled with this morning's "hangover" fog, that late nights don't suit me, despite the fact that they're alcohol-free!

Simon's supposed to be cooking us all breakfast but seems to be struggling with his back, an unfortunate casualty of rolling over to get out of bed. Again, I want to fulfil my role as a mum, so I find Deep Heat cream and painkillers, to try to at least alleviate the worst of his pain. But when it comes to the possibility of him seeing the doctor, I have to phone Sam and ask her if she can phone and speak to the surgery, as with my hearing the discussion would be almost impossible, particularly as he's not registered with them. Sam's good about it and also pops over, but I can't help but start to feel that now-familiar sense of displacement within my own family: it seems that once again I am handing over the role of the mother to my daughter, and I am nothing.

#

This evening brings a family outing to eat out, at my brother's suggestion. The idea's a grand one and everyone is keen to go, although I am extraordinarily tired. It's probably last night catching up with me and I don't want to be too tired to enjoy the christening, so I make the decision that if my brother and Simon stay on for a drink afterwards, I may come back home and settle myself early. Just thinking about it makes me feel like a party pooper though. All these years of family gatherings into the small hours and I've been at the centre of it all and now, I could just fall off the end of it without anyone even realising.

"I'll see how I go," I declare, making it sound like I'll let events decide, rather than the ache in my limbs, the roar in my ears and the confusion of my brain being the real reason for my retreat if it all gets too much.

The meal itself is very lovely: that part feels great, although I'm still peripheral to many of the conversations. Somehow, as I watch everyone, I'm reminded of the fact that extra actors filming crowd scenes are told to say "rhubarb, rhubarb" to sound like a babbling throng. If you can imagine the nonsensical rhubarb babble going on through a storm, or within the whoosh of a wind tunnel, then you're getting close enough to understanding my experience of the evening.

Some of Sam's friends are with us too and the baby takes her turn with all of us. At one point, one of Sam's friends is holding the baby, jiggling her about and whooshing her up and down, up and down. Suddenly, even with my hearing and my distance at the other end of the table, I hear a loud bang. We stop, just stop what we're doing, in that awful breath-held moment of silence before the baby begins to wail. Which, thankfully she does, lustily and extremely indignantly. It seems she wriggled, slipped down from the hands of her playmate and smacked her face on the edge of the table as she fell. The sound, that harsh, loud bang was the beautiful soft face of my grand-daughter cracking against the hard wood of the table – a reverberating echo of my own waking nightmares.

"These things happen" seems to be the sense around the table, but I can't adjust to their thinking. I can't get beyond this manifestation of my fears about all the possible harms that might come to this child, my beloved Evie. It's not tiredness which now leadens my limbs and sneaks away the words I want to use, it's an absolute anguish, made worse by the fact that Sam's friend, that clumsiest of all playmates, is laughing it off. Sure, I suspect that's probably nerves, or embarrassment, but it's not funny, it's just not funny. As the baby quietens and the rhubarb conversation moves back around the table, I watch as the shadow of a bruise starts to form under Evie's eye and around my very being.

#

Today, Christening day, Evie's eye seems a little less colourful which is probably just as well because my family are certainly colourful and high spirited enough! I too, want to dress up for the occasion, both for the event itself and for my own sake; this is the biggest outing and family event of my recovery so far. I wear my new dress, chosen with Frances, but know that I am not dressing up like old times when, instead of the trademark high heels of my 'old self' attire, I put on a pair of the tiniest heels I have ever worn. Despite the fact that they barely raise my heels an inch off the ground, I find it almost impossible to balance, so I attach myself firmly to my brother's arm for dear life as we set off for the church.

From the scatter of cars parked in the nearby car park to the little crowd in the church, it seems that all the invited family and friends have turned up, which is a grand mark of celebration and respect. The Christening itself is a pleasant, simple service, but very meaningful. I follow much of it from familiarity rather than actually hearing it, and of course the baby looks wonderful in her new-but-traditional Christening gown.

Afterwards, we all go back to the house. Although the day is a little cold, it's also very bright so we carry on with the plan for a finger buffet in the garden. Yesterday, when Simon, Julie, Joe, Ailbhe and myself had come round to help with the preparations, we'd decorated the garden with ribbons and bows. I'd worried slightly about them overnight in case they had become loose and soggy from the early dew, but they are fine, dancing in the slight breeze. I've spent many hours making these bows, in the dark wakefulness of my night-terrors, keeping my hands busy and my eyes occupied, fully focused on a useful task with a good, happy purpose, rather than being drawn to the shadowy rodents and other intangibles as they'd crept and flitted around me in the dark.

Normally, at a social gathering, I would be involved in some way, possibly the food preparation, or by circulating the drinks and refreshments. I suddenly grasp on to the thought that this is probably the first big family event where I don't have this role; it seems to be another thing the thief has taken that I hadn't yet missed or even been conscious of. Instead, I sit and watch as Sam's friends take the lead with the food, help to prepare the table or mix and serve drinks. I watch and ponder the idea, unsure if I am being protected or persecuted. Throughout the whole of these last six, horrible months, I don't think I've ever felt so left out or useless until this point, my first granddaughter's christening. I realise with a heart-sink that at no point has Sam asked, "Mum, do you think this, or that, is OK?" as she would have done in the past. My bows wave at me from the borders, on the sidelines like myself, making a silent contribution by dressing up the event, but not really participating; the friends have replaced me now.

#

My son and brother return to Ireland and I return to Sam's house. Each day I waken and think that today will be the day that I will be OK – I will just throw back the bed cover, get up and carry on as normal. But each morning the weight of the duvet remains rather more than I can actually lift, let alone throw and, as I stand to adjust myself and then stagger like an inebriate to the bathroom, I realise that it may not happen today; it may be tomorrow, yet tomorrow turns out to be just the same. My recovery seems based on that relentless hope of a better day tomorrow.

I deal with my morning ablutions trying to not to glimpse myself in the mirror, but of course it has to be done. My heart sinks and I cry some more. Lots of things make me cry but particularly this constant comparison of who I was before to who I am now, for myself and others.

I feel this most markedly when I get a peck on the cheek from my daughter and I see others get her warm hugs and of course I have to mention this to her. She ponders the thought for a moment, before replying calmly, "have you considered it may be that they are nicer people?"

So today, as all the other days, is spent trying to do what I can for myself but it is all just too much of an effort at times. It would be easy to give up, but something tells me I have to keep trying to get better. Constant prayers for help seem to be of no avail and neither are my prayers for release from this dreadful situation heard or answered, which I suppose means the answer is no. My first waking thought of the day is one of purpose - that this will be the day where things change and I maintain this thought as I stumble to the bathroom. However, by the time I've finished my ablutions, unwrapped my first incontinence pad of the day (if I don't count the one in the night) and staggered back to my room, my second thought of the day is that it's all hopeless.

#

The final big event of June and another signifier of my changing circumstances is that my last link with my old London life and the origins of my business comes to an end as my office there is closed down. This has meant that the remaining stock has had to be moved down here, to our new premises in St. Leonard's and I'm just so glad that I managed to get most of this arranged before my hearing got too bad.

Once again, where my business is concerned, I find myself humbled by those who aren't necessarily related to me who are willing to just help out to minimise stress and get things done for me. My old business partner, Ron, is one such person and this move, coming now when I've finally started to come to terms with (although naturally still fight against) the full extent of my cruel incapacities, almost has me on my knees with stress and exhaustion. My business has always been something I've relished, enjoyed building up and regarded as my ally in all of the other things I aimed to do in life, such as support my family and provide for my future but at this moment, as never before, the business suddenly feels like a huge responsibility, which I am almost too tired to face. It feels less of an ally and more like a stick that I'm being beaten with, something else of mine which the thief has also managed to get its hands on.

12. What the Thief Took

This seems to be the right kind of hiatus in which to consider this new person, coming out of the hospital, at least as a temporary reprieve from being in there, if not yet experiencing a reprieve from being ill.

And so, this is me. I'm still a person, a woman who's so much more than the sum of her symptoms, yet I'm so much less than the woman I used to be. The cunning thief, Viral Encephalitis has left gaping holes, made emmental of my brain, if you like. I guess it's no coincidence that there's "mental" within emmental, for this is how I seem with my unfinished sentences, my failure to read, write, speak with any kind of flow, let alone eloquence.

Then there's the tiredness. I find it hard to understand just the amount of hours in the day ... they are relentless and so tiring. But it's not like I'm doing anything, even the smallest thing, to wear myself out. But what the thief has taken in energy has been returned to me ten-fold in frustration: my persistent frustration at not being able to do even the simplest jobs and activities takes its toll.

Those around me carry on with their lives, even fitting in the extras like tending to me and the things I need. Take Sam, for example, with her home, her job and her baby and now a sick mother, an invalided mother; in-valid for sure. She just pulls in the energy from somewhere, rallies her resources like an army and soldiers on. Just watching her exhausts me whilst I recline in the bed.

Sounds comfortable doesn't it? But it's not all it should be, the luxury of a lie-in, of the chance to rest, to recover. Yes, I recline in the bed, but I'm as uncomfortable as the legendary princess with the pea ... because of course with my continence and self-control being whisked away by the thief, there is a very real pee issue here. I'm uncomfortable in my body and its functions. Pads are intimately intrusive and I cannot, will not, rely on them. I'm conscious of the smell of myself, not just the stench of my sickness, which I feel still lingers around me like an exclusive, expensive perfume, but the smell of my incontinence, the very real eau-de-toilet, as it were.

This shouldn't be something I have in common with my grand-daughter but, here we are. Each of us lie in our own effluence until, in her case, the matter is dealt with – swiftly, competently, with a smile, soft wipes, talc and tenderness.

Here our similarities stop. My matter is dealt with through my exhausted, exasperated wobbling to the bathroom for attention from my own, unco-ordinated hands. Of course, unco-ordinated hands make for clumsy movements which, when combined with dubious balance and soiled pads, means half an hour spent in a way which is not for the faint-hearted. I spend more time cleaning up *after* myself than I do cleaning myself up, if you see what I mean, as I have none of the attributes needed to deal with the issue competently. It's messy, it's time-consuming and it's unfair. I spend a considerable time "sorting myself out" before I can finally bag up my soiled pads, just as Sam bags up the baby's nappies.

Sometimes, after the rigours of my clean-up campaign, which may also involve having to shower again and then ensuring my new pad is in situ with no potential for leaks, I might forget about my previous pad, forget to bag it up, before disposing of it in the bathroom bin. This is wrong, of course it is and I have to be reminded, time after time, that this just isn't the thing to do. I don't mean to forget, but there it is. The thief took my control as well as my means to manage myself, leaving me a problem of my own bodily making to sort out: I have to deal with the problem, no talc or tenderness, just tears and tissues, endless tears and tissues.

#

The thief has also taken my time. I don't just mean those precious months I've spent in hospital or even the relentless days of "recovery" I'm spending now. I mean MY time, my prime-of-life time. Ok, so that might be a cliché but it's my cliché and I've been denied it. I had my plans, my third age ambitions, but now?

In some corners of my past I have sometimes wondered how our lives as a family might pan out ... constantly praying for no illness to befall us so that we just die of old age, after a full life, when our time comes – from the oldest to the youngest of us. It's something of a shock then, to find that my time may have been upon me, and that my best times, my best capabilities, the shape and sensibilities that make up my very soul have now been taken. I never expected that I would be first to be stricken with an illness that would catapult me from 57 to feeling like 70. I'm not without hope, of course, for I do see a lot of nifty 70 year olds about but at the moment, I'm not one of them ... they are more capable than me, in truth I have more niff than nifty about me since the thief struck.

I'm conscious of losing my time in the sense of what came before. From the heartbreak of not knowing my own child, to the annoying lack of recall of what's said to me ... every emotion in between can be attached to the time I've lost through the thief's ransacking of my memory, of its content as well as its capacity.

And of what's to come? Who's to know how far this theft of my time extends? I'm supposed to be a grandmother, fulfil the role with vigour, anticipation and humour, to enjoy my grandchild's growing up time. It can't be right that her growing up time has collided with my own slowing up time ... I'm at a standstill whilst she races on. Of course we do have some parallels, marvellously inconvenient ones, such as our shared, wobbly way of walking, our pad-dependent toileting and our inarticulate communications where we can't say what we mean or even mean what we say. And for how long will we remain like this, my pause, her progression? Sooner or later, she will be writing, reading and speaking fluently, coherently, whilst I remain pen poised to produce only scribbles, mechanically reading and then forgetting what I've read, planning to say something important, only to forget exactly where the thought was taking me, what I was going to ...?

#

I'm conscious too, that my sense of humour also seems to have been stolen away whilst I was sleeping. It even seems to have abandoned me even when I am on good form - I can't remember when I had a good smile, never mind a good laugh. Who said "laughter is the best medicine?" I wish that person could visit with me, add a splash of fun to my recovery. The trouble is, even if I can hear the joke, most of the time I just can't compute it, can't process the nuances of the language, of the timing, especially not in time to laugh alongside others. Comedy's all about the timing right? I'm so far behind that one now, it's almost hilarious.

As a result, life seems to have become very serious, there is little fun - an occasional joke with my sister on my adapted phone but even that is limited. People don't converse any more than they have to and when I try to join in I usually only get the gist of the conversation which, as hard as I try, I just can't piece together the blanks of because I have too many blanks of my own.

Sure, I can ask for it to be repeated … but when I do? I get told it doesn't matter – but of course it does - I didn't bloody well hear and I want to. I want to share the joke, not *be* the joke.

#

Now, I know I'll talk at length about my hearing loss – something the thief took so stealthily that even now, all this time later, none of the medics can really tell me for sure whether my hearing loss is due to the thief's action, or the medications on their VE damage limitation quest. It's no matter really, I suppose. To me, either way, my hearing is something that the thief is ultimately responsible for taking.

One of the reasons why I find my deafness so isolating is that my hearing used to involve me in so many things, so I now feel robbed many times over, of my hearing and my involvement in richer, wider, fun activities. Until I became ill, I sang in choral groups, first in Wimbledon 25 years ago, then joining this one soon after moving to East Sussex. Some of the women are marvelous, particularly Yvonne and Mary, they're both great for the regular coffee and a chat. Yvonne's son is our musical director, so even in the early days of being released from hospital she has always kept me up to date with all that I'm missing out on. Mary and I have always just clicked, right since I joined the group, sharing jokes and ideas about our performances. There's never been any question in their minds, or mine, that I'd be rejoining the group, ready to pick up with the practices for either of the two concerts we give every year: Christmas and summer.

It's when I'm about to go back to the singing group, at the beginning of May 2008, when my hearing really starts to fade. At rehearsal I receive a lovely warm welcome from nearly everyone but almost at once there's a problem with me being at the practice; I'm still weak and can't stand for the duration of the whole rehearsal. Of course, singing is about being upright and breathing deeply so I'm told, quite rightly, that I can't sit ... I can't sit and sing. But as I'm standing, my hearing starts to play tricks. I strain to catch the music but I just can't hear the tunes, pick up the melodies. Oh I can hear noise alright, but that's all it is, tuneless, loud noise, so bad that the melody is lost. I think maybe it's because I'm overdoing it: by being there, by trying to stand for so long, by surrounding myself with loud, vibrant voices. The truth is though, that this is the moment that the impact of the thief on my hearing is really starting to show.

I still attend the concert, later in the summer but by then the cost of the ticket is completely wasted on me. I follow the programme and Sam tells me what they are singing. If I know the song, I try to imagine it, listen to it in my head rather than from the full choir standing in front of me. I know where I would have been standing, what part would have been mine in the harmony, but I can't even hear where they are, let alone join in.

I can't describe how much I want to be able to join in. It's like that childhood feeling of not being picked, not being old enough or, worse, capable enough to be involved with the more fun activities of the others. I'm completely on the outside of this. I've always found music emotionally arousing, yet this time I can't stop the tears because *the music can't touch me*. I can't experience those notes which tingle the back of your neck with a shiver or draw a tear of joy and I have no idea if I'll ever be able to again. The tears just keep coming, until the choir appear to be standing in a sea-mist. I know that this moment's not the time for those tears or fears, but I know now that another part of my life has been taken from me: there is no music, no rhythm in my soul, no dance in my heart.

#

It's not until over a year after losing my hearing that anyone is able to come close to revealing any understanding of how I feel about this loss. We're all at one of my sister's parties and I'm hating every minute of it, because for me this party is a snapshot which highlights everything I've lost to the thief ...

We're sitting around a table again and instead of enjoying my meal I'm watching masticating mouths full of food as I try to lip-read to keep up with conversations, oh joy, such is my effort to keep up with table-time banter. Meanwhile, in the recess of my mind, I'm worried about my continence. I'm sitting here hoping with all my heart that my Tenas have protected me and that I won't stand up with a wet seat on my trousers. My body, already stiff, moves surreptitiously, cautiously, fearing the shame of a leak, of leaving a wet patch that is mine on a chair which isn't. These are the intruding thoughts whilst others enjoy the company, yet I can't join in with the chat, the banter; the family jokes are lost, wasted on me. Then, as well as missing the jokes, I can't hear the speeches. In the dim light of the party it's hard to lip-read them instead, so it's all like pictures going on around me, with a background noise but no discernable sounds.

And it's your typical Irish party, so the singers, everyone's daughters, nieces and friends are here, belting out their songs. Everyone's joining in ... except me. I'm not even sure I remember the words to the old songs, this ingrained soundtrack of my childhood. Even if I try, I don't know where I am to join in as I can't hear the tune or the rhythm and I don't trust my voice, my loud, unpractised voice; I can't hear how I sound so I have no idea what kind of noise comes out.

I hold it all together for as long as I can, but by about 11 pm I've had enough. It's too difficult trying to be strong, trying to be 'together', trying to be as 'better' as everyone wants me to be. I come to get some quiet time in my room and of course each of my kindly sisters comes to see where I am.

"You might as well be downstairs as here, you'd be better off," one tells me but I can't work that one out. I've only just made the decision that I'd be better off on my own for a while but now it seems my decision isn't right either.

I'm wracked with sobs until my brother comes to find me. He's just arrived and, for completely different reasons and after a long period of deafness, he's had a cochlea implant, which has completely changed his life. He sits with me awhile and is understanding, but it's short lived.

"I know what a lonely place you are in," he says, simply.

And that's the crux of it. He doesn't trot out the platitudes about asking people to speak up, he doesn't offer anything other than his absolute understanding, which gives me more strength than anything. After a time, once my eyes are a little less red, I am able to join them for the rest of the party, anxious to regain even the smallest part of these losses, a little company amongst the loneliness.

#

And it's true that in there, amongst the losses of hearing, the personality, the patience and the humour, is the absence of my ability to experience pleasure. I can still manage this within certain remits and, as I get stronger, so too does my capacity to find pleasure in the smallest things, such as my garden (although absolute, relaxed pleasure in this takes a long while to arrive thanks to the sinister movements I catch from the corner of my eyes, the perceived rats with their accompanying terrors which stalk me for such a long time). Pleasure is one of the losses I am working hard to claw back. Once I wrestle my positivity away from the pervading fears, then this too will be something I regain.

Family gatherings are of course pleasant, more-so when I consider that not so long back when I didn't even recognise or feel I knew close loved ones, members of my family. Some of this I have managed to regain and take pleasure in. And I do try to take pleasure in such gatherings even if, as an experience, they look far more pleasant than they actually are.

Where there is lots of talk, it's just impossible to keep up and I miss things or have to wade in to ask what they are talking about. Most usually the first response is "have you got your hearing aids in?" This is a popular misconception, because only people with certain kinds of hearing difficulty have the same instant relief from hearing aids as a spectacle wearer does from putting on those glasses. Yes, I have my hearing aids in and switched on, but sometimes they are as useful to me as a blindfold and just as confusing and disorientating!

I try to take pleasure in conversation but it's still difficult to keep up with more than one person. I lose the visual help of lip reading when they twist round to speak with each other, turning away from me, so it becomes like my limited memory of being on a mobile phone with a bad signal when you keep losing the voice on the other end.

The conversations continue around me, fragmented snippets reach me, fractured by distractions and interruptions - this is all hard work and not very enjoyable. I have to pay close attention to facial expressions to know whether this is a joke, to know that someone's laughing rather than in pain.

I ask what they are talking about I'm told, for example: "he's an Irish journalist, you wouldn't know him" ... however I try there is little result, conversation's too difficult all round so people move off, drift away from me. So I spectate, on the outside looking in, trying to gain pleasure in just being here. But I'm not here, really. OK, so the thief didn't take the whole of me but the bits that are left just don't feel like they are living. There's nowhere that I fit: I've lost chunks of my past, my future is beset with limitations and my participation in the present is decidedly negligible.

#

As such, in light of what the thief took, I sometimes wonder if I am of less value than the rest of my family, that I should have succumbed to this virus and suffered the consequences of being left with so little and improving so very slowly, as I am doing?

It seems the Encephalitis has the ability to rampage through, damaging the brain, wiping out all the unconscious protective barriers we build up over the years and rendering us, in my experience: juvenile; uneducated; vulnerable and fearful - all the things we tend to mask in normal existence. For such a thief, it's the ultimate prize, the crown jewels: my "normal" has been taken. I am what is left.

13. Someone Around Here Needs Therapy

It's the first of July today and I find I'm now counting each new month according to a different timeline, not only since the VE (now month seven) but also since the deafness. It's now been two long months since I went deaf and that's a long time to be cut off and isolated from a world I'd been trying to re-acquaint myself with. It's also an eternity to be spending having to adjust, trying to find the things which will make life easier, less lonely. I guess in a perfect world, if the same situation had arisen there would have been a useful X, Y and Z of routes to follow to ease things, help me to find my way. However I also suppose the VE wouldn't have risen at all, if the world was *that* perfect.

Sadly though, the world is less than perfect and what's more, although on my own isolated plane most of the time I'm currently actually occupying the physical space of someone else's world and there-in lies the problem, as some of the possible solutions to the hearing are less easy to resolve.

Very occasionally, I can hold conversations on my mobile or house phone, which is liberating to say the least. So, I ask Sam if I can get a phone with a loud speaker, to use as her house phone. However, she tells me she will have to speak to Simon about it and suggests instead that I should bring the phone with a loudspeaker from my house. The trouble with that suggestion is that I need that whilst I am there, and of course I am trying to be there when possible to build up towards independent living. Eventually, in desperation I buy a handset for Sam's, complete with a loudspeaker that I should be able to use. Unfortunately, it needs to be set up first and, because there isn't the same urgency for them as there is for me to get it done and I'm not tech savvy enough to do it myself, it remains sitting on my table, unplugged and useless, a bit like me. Trust me, if I could do this myself, I would. Instead I sit here, thwarted by the VE, the deafness and now the technology!

#

I'm not particularly computer literate either, but I do manage most things on it, like I can use it at work. The thing is though that I don't seem to have the time, much less the patience, to just sit in front of it and learn how to do new things, so I'm limited to the few tasks I have remembered or have been re-shown. I'd like to be able to do more and the best way to learn is to have a specific thing to need to do and have someone show you how to do it. My laptop at home has a different screen to Sam's home computer and this throws me completely: I'm so used to using it one way and now have to learn a new way, but no-one has time to spare – either to show me or to let me monopolise the computer for the significant amount of time it would take me to find out how to do certain things for myself.

Today, I really need to get on Sam's PC and find a list of approved complementary therapists for some neck treatment, for a niggle which has been troubling me for over a week now. I asked the GP about a chiropractor and his answer was a distinct "no" so I need to find a gentler complementary therapy. Each time I ask for some help to conduct a search on the computer to see if there's anyone locally, it doesn't seem to be the right time. Sam says we can do it on Monday, when she's off.

#

I waken to my usual tears but try to shake off the gloom with the realisation that it's Monday, so instead I start to build a happy anticipation that we'll be getting on the computer to find someone who can help my neck and hopefully my ears too whilst we're there.

First though, there's the usual Monday routine of spending time at my business, which we do for a couple of hours, until both the baby and myself are too tired and fretful to continue. Today, on the way home it's necessary to stop off in town as Sam wants to return some cushions and run a few errands. By the time we're home and have had lunch, I sit in the garden with the baby whilst Sam pops to the local chemist to pick up my prescription.

When Sam gets back, the computer is duly fired up, ready for action but first she has to look at her e-mails, something to do with a friend's bath which has been leaking for several months. This seems to be something of a priority for a reason that I just can't fathom. I'd pace the garden if I had the energy and the stride (pacing is not actually the purposeful activity it sounds when sticks are involved) because, as everyone knows by now, I am a patient by label only, no longer by personality. By the time Sam does come back out to the garden, the baby needs a feed which, quite rightly, is a main priority. I remove myself (and my itching tongue) from the situation by going to do juicing for all of us, losing myself to the whirr and spin of the juicer. By the time each of these events is completed, Simon is home so they take Evie for a stroll in the late afternoon sun whilst I walk in the opposite direction for my acupuncture appointment. When I return, it's too late for computer time because the day's highlights of Wimbledon are on the TV.

This sort of thing makes me feel that my hearing is not a priority to them and that they would be happy I stay deaf or go home. I feel uncharitable thinking this about my own family, but justified in equal measures: I'm shocked by the person I'm becoming but can't help feeling glad that I want to assert myself, that I don't have to be so helpless, so passive. What I don't want to do though, is rock the boat, so I take myself off to bed early. Frances is coming soon, Frances will understand.

#

My plans for Frances take on the same form as for my brother and son during last month's christening visit. I'm hoping to move back home for Frances to stay with me, to give Sam and Simon some much needed alone time and, in truth, to give myself the same thing (albeit under the genial, watchful eye of my sister).

As usual Carol and Gordon help me prepare the house and garden, but I do note for myself that I too am able to contribute a little more to the preparations this time around, including a little levity from time to time. This stay will be good for all of us, I'm sure.

#

Of course, real life doesn't stop, even for the auspicious weeks of my sister's visit. I've been waiting so long for my appointment with the Clinical Psychologist ... I honestly can't remember how far back it was when the neurologist managed to get a word in edge-wise through my blubbering woes, to suggest that it might be a good step in helping to cope with the emotional and physical state the VE has left me with. So, another waiting list although on this occasion we were specifically told that my wait would be longer than most because it was considered important that I see someone who specialises in Encephalitis and ABI.

Imagine my mixed feelings then, when the first appointment letter finally arrived and I realised that it was scheduled within those first few days of Frances's stay. Of course, I needn't have worried – her response was just the same as for the audiologist appointment during her last visit: "that's fine, I can drive you, save you the taxi fare and I can be there … you know, just be there."

And so here we are on our way to the 11 am appointment. I know this building, I've passed it many times but I don't think I really knew what went on here. Despite my own training, both as a seating technician and as a counsellor, all those years of working alongside physicians as well as vulnerable people, I'm finding myself hand-sweaty nervous about now being amongst those "vulnerable" ones. I'm not sure what I expect to find inside, but the waiting room is clean and respectable. I hobble in on my sticks and Frances's arm, feeling as scared as a five year old going to the dentist for the first time.

As we sit, I keep reminding myself that, as a qualified counsellor, I know the drill but somehow knowing this doesn't prepare me for having to acknowledge that I have an emotional problem, as a result of a physical condition. Frances is a comforting presence and I'm glad she's here, but it doesn't make me feel any less worthless, passive and so very unable for this session. My mouth is as dry as my hands are clammy. I try to distract myself by wondering which of the closed doors the miraculous help will happen behind.

My name is called and Frances nudges me. The psychologist seems friendly enough as she introduces herself and we walk to her room, where a student is sitting at the side of the room, wearing a nervy kind of professionalism. The psychologist asks if I have any objections to the student's presence and I don't … I can just about remember what it's like to be learning about this stuff myself, so she's welcome and if she can learn anything from me then, well that's all to the good for someone then, isn't it?

To my shock, mingled with an "oh well, if not here, then where?" kind of relief, the moment I am seated in the chair and the psychologist starts speaking to me, so kindly, about the reasons for the intervention, I start to cry. Ah no, I mean sob. I am sobbing my heart and my story out to this captive clinician and hapless student. I have no means to stop and I know that I'm being a "classic" patient in need of emotional support, because I'm doing what most people going to a therapist try to do: I'm launching, on a tide of my own tears, into the overwhelming tempest of my existence. I sob and stutter and don't come up for air throughout, except for the shortest time at the beginning, when she stops me just long enough to deliver the confidentiality clause. After this, it's no holds barred and I spill my grievances about the dramatic effects of the Encephalitis on my old self, my grim thoughts, nightly prayers and of course my overwhelming anxiety and sadness about the effect of my illness on my relationship with my daughter, whilst all the time the psychologist scribbles in her pad and places tissue after tissue into my shaking hands.

At the end, she has two pieces of news for me, one of which is no surprise whilst the other so shocks me so that I'm speechless for the first time since setting foot into her office. Firstly, she tells me that my current state of mind is because I'm in an adjustment period. Of course that's no surprise at all, it's what everyone's been telling me and what I have figured out for myself: but this transition from old me to new me doesn't feel like "just" adjustment, the word *adjustment* itself suggests flexibility, whereas my situation has a permanence and I can't adjust to the new me whilst I'm still trying to find the old one, wherever she's gone.

And the shocking news? She tells me kindly and gently that I am her first Encephalitis patient. So, all my waiting for someone with experience was a waste of time, a complete waste of my time! Really? Yes, really. I'm stunned: how much farther down this road of "adjustment" would I be now without that extra wait which was, I hasten to add, placed upon me, not sought by me? To say I feel slightly let down would be a minor understatement and, understatement being the current order of things, I lapse into my first silence. Gently, professionally, she takes the opportunity to tell me she's organising another appointment for the following week, but this next one will take place at the rehabilitation unit at the hospital. And so, it's the end of the session and I come out from behind the closed door where I'm not sure any kind of miracle has happened. I make my way back to the waiting room to meet my sister, who I am so, so glad is here.

#

Part of the plan during Frances's stay is for us to go down to Dorset to visit our Uncle, the last surviving member of our father's family. We're not planning on taking the train as Frances has volunteered to drive. Now, I'm trying not to be obsessively anxious about this, but although I have confidence in her driving, I remain terrified of being away from home and struggle with my confidence in my own ability to cope with the trip.

However, that aside, although this trip is closely-related to family reasons, I'm also looking forward to it as the chance for a short break, my only chance for a little holiday since the thief snatched away my holiday plans earlier in the year. Frances is fun to be with and, in truth, I'm also gaining confidence or, as I think of it, a false-confidence that comes from having a companion, a back-up person with me, much of which stems from her own self-assurance about the drive. In truth, I'm finding her enthusiasm for the trip to be quite infectious.

After a slightly false start because the sun roof won't open, despite the intervention of the local garage, we decide to get going. There's probably a joke somewhere about not attempting to be topless at our age anyway, but I'm getting a little too anxious for jokes and merry-making. This transport delay is slightly akin to my experiences with the hospital transport system and I'm finding my heart-rate rising as a fist-clenching, jaw-setting anxiety starts to creep its way into my blood.

Thankfully, Frances is happy to set off regardless as, although it's hot, we're unlikely to want the roof down as it's extremely windy, particularly when you factor in the wind-rush from those faster roads. Oh yes, those faster roads. In the hospital transport and Sam's car, toddling around town, I'd forgotten about the raw speed and closeness of "proper" traffic. Out here on the A roads and the motorways, the blur of the other traffic shakes my senses. I try to keep my anxieties to myself, but find myself dry-mouthed and fidgety, despite the pain in my body. We're part of the flow and roar of the traffic and I don't like it one bit.

We stop at a service station near Southampton, which has a public picnic area. After the strange sensation of being in the rush of the traffic, I seem to be in a "sea legs" situation and find myself slightly more wobbly than usual as I adjust to being back on solid ground! We enjoy our salad and a cup of tea for about an hour and then, just like those early days of being at Sam's and having to tackle journeys up and down the stairs, it feels like I'm just about adjusted and then it's time for the next leg of the journey.

This time, the roads are slightly more pleasant, taking us through the verdant New Forest, where, like a child, I distract myself from feeling ill by looking out for the horses. Of course, with all the other creatures I regularly "see" in my peripheral vision, actually identifying the ponies is quite tricky, but it all serves as a useful distraction until we thankfully arrive in Wareham about 5pm.

And so to our holiday accommodation – or not, as it happens. On arrival at the little pub hotel where I've often stayed, I'm faced with not only new proprietors, but also the fact the place is totally full. Literally, although accommodating by nature, it seems they don't have any room for us. I feel my anxiety level once again rising, my worth suddenly coming into question: Frances has handled the drive, I'm handling this bit, yet I've messed it up, messed it up completely. I'm not sure what expression I'm wearing by this time, but I can feel my disappointment tingle across my face and I realise I don't know what to do next. Thankfully though, this extremely pleasant new owner suddenly points across the road, towards another pub B & B in a little quay on the other side of the road. She's also describing another alternative, a hotel a mile away.

I stumble back out to update Frances with our options, trying not to sound flustered although a straight swap of anxiety, from the no accommodation situation to the dilemma of having to make a decision, takes place somewhere within me. However, with Frances alongside it's easy, no dithering at all as I assume Frances's confidence as a cloak of my own - in an instant it seems we have opted for the quay-side pub as neither of us really wants another car journey and this alternative, overlooking the river with the boats bobbing up and down, people fishing and a car park which seems to be a meeting place for walkers, is something close to picture-postcard perfect.

Our decision's the right one; they not only have availability, they also have their luxury accommodation of a house adjoining the pub available. Delighted, we book in and move our bags into the house. Now 'luxury' is a subjective word and, to be honest (which of course I am, intolerably so) as I look around our home for the next couple of days, luxury is not a word I would have used to describe the accommodation, furnishings, decoration and all. However, it offers a sanctuary from the journey, a hiatus from the rigours of my relentless search for recovery and the bizarre "normal" routine that comes with it and of course, particularly for Frances after the long drive, it's a peaceful place to rest. To that end, Frances and I agree that it's very nice and that we're more than happy with the way we've completed the first part of our mission.

#

The next mission is to find Bonnett's Lane, my uncle's address, which we do easily as it is less than 10 minutes away. We are greeted by a pleasant, but clearly very professional lady who takes us through the security drill, signs us in and checks not only who we are seeing but whether we are carrying any alcohol. The fact she even asks gives me quite an unexpected shiver of naughtiness as in reality, since the VE, I am the least naughty person I know!

We're led to our uncle's room. The remnant memories of my past career, which still float by on occasions are enhanced by the sights and smells of this residence. I used to visit all sorts of nursing homes, care institutions, day centres and residential homes. Despite thirty years of doing that I can't recall too much but I know that my instinctive, immediate impression of this place is by subconscious comparison to all those others I've ever visited and that this impression is favourable. There's no smell of urine, no stench of neglect and all those we pass, both staff and residents, look happy.

Walking past open doorways you can catch the signs, you see, by spotting how the day-to-day interactions and routines are being played out. All the staff we pass seem respectful towards their residents. This has always been important to me as a professional, but since being a patient it has become one of those things that I could be border-line obsessive about. Despite memories I've lost, I've retained vivid, awful ones of all the horrid situations I've seen people in: sitting, waiting, just waiting – be it for care assistants, meals on wheels, medics, any kind of contact with the outside world. This memory loop is one which made me determined I was not going to be seeing out my remaining days plopped in front of a blaring 40" screen, just waiting.

So I'm watchful as we trail the corridors. I'm sure I don't know what I'd do, what kind of attention and chaos I'd cause if I happened to see something less than respectful, less than kind, less than caring and I'm slightly on edge with both this and the anticipation of how our uncle will be. But I see nothing except signs of happiness (and believe me, I do not wear rosy coloured spectacles about these places) so I'm greatly reassured. As the door opens to our uncle's room, my reassurance is complete; he's delighted with his surprise visit and we're overjoyed to find him in good form. He's clean, cared for and looking so well. I feel for him with a tangible pain, being so vulnerable, so reliant on all of this outside assistance, yet he's good-natured and happy about it, so I too must be happy for him.

We spend about an hour and a half with him. He's chatty enough and content, he clearly feels at home here. Between us, Frances and I arrange the flowers we've brought him. We create a vase of flowers with cheery beaming sunflowers, his favourites, and Stargazer lilies. I'm filled with a sense of cheer and contentment, both for him and because of him and, although these places can often be miserable and maudlin, I find myself feeling optimistic in a way that I haven't for some time which even saying goodbye, which I don't like, cannot diminish.

As we head back to our accommodation we stop in the pub for dinner. It's a real novelty for me and I'm not feeling nearly as self-conscious as I usually do, like at the christening meal last month. Frances and I are totally relaxed and enjoy exchanging our views about the menu. In the end, we decide on "Black Rock" or as Frances knows it, "Hot Stone Cuisine." It's quite innovative and, having been isolated from trends for so long, I find it fascinating. The meat comes raw, on this hot stone: the idea is you cut off bite size pieces, then cook and eat them individually; the main piece is cooking on the stone all the time. Frances tries the chicken and I indulge myself with rib-eye steak. It's a real treat and I, who have struggled in the recent past with managing basic cutlery, adapt to the hot stone process with a comparative ease which elevates both my humour and my confidence.

Over dinner, we chat about our uncle, both of us happy to have seen him looking so well and contented, and then we discuss the meal, agreeing that the baked potato was the best ever and our salad the perfect accompaniment to the whole thing. I feel like a proper part of this conversation, I can contribute ideas and opinions and know that there's nothing that will be misunderstood and, importantly, that I'm well placed to avoid misunderstandings myself. Between my hearing aids and Frances's professional role, where she is mindful to stay face-on to me as she talks so that I can watch her lips and face to support my understanding of her words, I feel almost like my old self, relaxing, chewing the fat (in all ways) with my sister. I want to hold on to this feeling, keep it safe under my pillow so that I wake up with it tomorrow.

After paying, we retire to the house, or rather I do; Frances wants to take in the night air. I'm exhausted so she goes off for her stroll whilst I stay put. I have the creeping, cold sensation that somehow I must have already put my good feeling safely under the pillow for tomorrow because it's deserted me now. Within moments of Frances leaving me on my own, the anxieties and fears creep in. I can't be so nervous about being alone, it's ridiculous, I chastise myself. Yet I am. I am.

I try to read to distract myself. I manage a bit but the ghouls in my peripheral vision have moved their cases in too and distract me immensely. I decide to send a few text messages instead, something which really requires focus. But of course, I have no signal. I move to the window and watch the boats, barely moving on the slick, black water. I've taken out my hearing aids and so, without the din of the restaurant, the street and everything but the voices of fear in my head and the whoosh of my ears, it's surprisingly peaceful and scenic. I'm still scared though. Frances arrives back and I immediately become nonchalant about the time alone, no, no troubles, all fine. Our final act of the day is a crossword, of course a challenge for me but being with Frances makes it fun, like a game, it doesn't feel like a direct confrontation to my limited capabilities. Actually, it makes me smile ... there's that saying about never going to sleep on a cross word, but here we are, Frances and I, sharing a crossword before bed. I'm aware, as we finally settle to sleep, that this is one of my very best, good days so far.

#

Of course, all good things and that ... today my body is on pay-back for yesterday's exertions. I remain in bed, my body aching, head pounding whilst Frances gets up and goes off to do her yoga down by the river. I stay laying here, waiting for my body to calm a little. Unlike last night, I'm not really scared on my own at the moment, I'm used to daytime alone time at Sam's and, without fear, my body can at least relax and rest a little more easily.

Eventually though, I do rally myself to get up and open the blinds. I can see Frances, a silhouette of postures against the already sunny backdrop. I try to mirror some of the poses she's doing, but to do so requires a balance that I just don't have. The only ones I have a vague chance of being successful with are the lying down ones but of course as soon as I lie down, I can't see out of the window to follow her movements. It strikes me quite humorous and I share it with Frances when she comes back and she laughs too, with me, not at me.

#

It turns out lucky we're starting the day in a good humoured way for we go into the pub for breakfast and immediately nickname the whole establishment "Fawlty Towers." After last night's feast, we each decide not to have full English, instead I choose bacon and tomato, Frances wants tomato and egg and we'd both like tea and toast, please. The Chinese girl who's standing beside us pleasantly and patiently noting the order just does not understand this aberration from the main menu and has to go and get her manager, who is clearly not happy about having to get involved. He obviously leaves his personality and manners at his desk before approaching our table, to check what it is we want to eat. He checks three times in total, each time relaying it back to us incorrectly. Part of me is starting to feel extremely frustrated, but one glance at Frances and instead, I want to start giggling. Just as he seems to have grasped what we actually do want, his attention is distracted by a motor biker, clearly identifiable by his leathers and the helmet under his arm, who comes into the pub smiling asking for a coffee.

The manager's brush-off is brusque and clearly off-pat. "We don't open till eleven." A glance at the clock shows there are ten minutes to go. It appears that as guests in the luxury accommodation we have certain privileges, you see. A glance back to the motor biker reveals that weary expression which tells you he's in a coffee-or-die kind of zone. He and the manager are eyes-locked, jaws set, so Frances intervenes:

"Give him a coffee," she orders "and charge it to me."

The look the manager gives her is priceless; this could be a real stand-off situation, but instead of getting more annoyed, we find ourselves laughing and the biker man beams at us, so the manager can do nothing but move off to fulfil everyone's order! This is a dignified moment for two daring don't-mess-with-us Irish ladies of a certain age, or at least would be, if we could stop giggling.

Fawlty Towers frivolities over, we then load the car and head back to find Uncle Joe sitting in the dining room, showered and ready since 8am, waiting for us. We enjoy a couple of hours, until almost 2pm before we have to say goodbye one last time to him. Before leaving town though, we indulge one last holiday moment with a walk into town. We visit a few little art shops, always my favourite kind of past-time and I buy four pretty hat boxes, white with delicate red roses, from a charity shop as a small treat to myself.

We decide to leave Wareham about 3pm and plan to have dinner on the way and perhaps enjoy one more holiday meal just like last night. At some point around Southampton we're both feeling peckish so we agree to stop at the next service station, which happens to be a Little Chef. The menu's not too imaginative although the salads we're served do actually require a bit of imagination to see them as such! We deal with it affably enough though, Frances and I, but managed more with a tired pragmatism than the humour of this morning's breakfast mayhem; as far as we're concerned, the holiday spirit has given way to fatigue for both of us and this meal is now just something to keep us going.

I find it hard getting back into the car for the last leg of the journey. My body is starting to roar with pain and stiffness but it's a necessary pain. I've faced lots of fears over these two days: the fear of being away from home, away from Sam, Simon and Evie; the fear of the trip highlighting my abilities and lack of abilities; managing the drive with the sensory overload and the pain, stiffness and sore skin. Not to mention, of course, the damn incontinence, which brings with it a desperate need to always know where I can go to sort myself out. This worry's always significantly there and although I knew I was going to visit our uncle in a nursing home where (of all places) there would certainly be facilities and understanding, that was always going to be the last kind of place where I'd want to be succumbing to the urgency and embarrassment of those kinds of symptoms.

But the last part of the journey's not really so bad and as we arrive back into Hastings on the coastal road, a walk along the seafront to stretch our cramped legs seems to be the perfect end to the day. I struggle out of the car, bent and stiff but am no sooner starting to stretch out a little than it begins to rain. I'm so mindful of my herbalist's warning that I must stay out of the wind and not get wet that I decide to return to the car and wait for Frances, so I fold myself back into the passenger seat once more. I'm not sure if this action comes under the label of fearful or careful, but either way it marks my return back to the "normal" routine, which I guess generally falls between the two at the best of times.

#

It's Friday, 18th July and it's the final full day of Frances's stay, so we spend an easy day together, both in the house and by popping out and about down the town. A short while after we arrive home from town, Frances decides to take a final walk around the block, before her long journey back. Whilst she's gone, I find myself looking around my home, because I am now, much more, regarding it as my home. I'm conscious that I'm at something of a crossroads. I've been so happy here, in my home with all my recent visitors and to return, back to the routine of fearful and careful in the context of Sam's house seems to present itself as something of a backward step, especially as I think I've really done well these past weeks, including these past few days with the trip.

I'm so busy mulling this over that I don't realise an hour has passed and that Frances has texted me. Her text tells me she has gone to the seafront to walk some more but not to worry, she'll get a taxi back. Although this is a bit of a deviation to the plan, I find myself surprisingly relaxed about it, her thoughtful text really helping me not to panic about being alone, not knowing where she's got to or when she'll be back. With this condition, the way I am "normally", there's no space for adjustment to arrangements but here I am, not completely relaxed but able, to a certain extent, to go with the flow. Yes, I've come a long way these last few weeks, I think.

#

The next day, Saturday, Frances leaves as planned and I mooch about the house, my house. A strange feeling that I can only describe as a positive tension seems to be invading me and I can't quite explain it.

I'm still trying to cope with, let alone define how I'm feeling, when Sam and her mother-in-law call to pick me up. We're going to a concert that some of my choir colleagues have invited me to, as they are performing. Perhaps this is behind the feeling? The event proves to be torturous in a very contradictory way, to be honest. After all, I can't hear and have little idea of what is going on, yet it is good to catch up with others when it's over.

As we get into the car, Sam turns to me and asks "where to?" Without a hint of dither or indecision, I reply "home" and I mean home, my home. After all, lots of my necessities are there from the stay with Frances - my medication and creams, so I'd need to get them anyway. At one point it crosses my mind that perhaps I could just spend the late evening there and return to Sam's to sleep, but I think this creeping tension since this morning is to do with a realisation that there are no half-measures about this; the time has come to be at home. By spending the night at home, it will be much easier for me emotionally to stay put – I can just take my sleeping tablet and go to bed. For someone so continually plagued by such paralysing indecision, I feel surprisingly clear in my head about this, almost to the point of giddiness, if that's not a complete contradiction: I've decided I'll do it and I'll do it, enough said.

Sam's kind and reassuring, immediately offering me lots of options in the event that I might change my mind. I must call her at any time, I must call if I want a lift, I mustn't get a cab. She's adamant about this and obviously wants to cover all bases in the event of everything from a simple change of mind to a major calamity. Although she means well, it confuses me to get so many options. Finally I find myself responding:

"OK, but just take me home, don't talk about it."

So here I am, it's July 19th, seven months after being taken ill and four months after being discharged for that "fortnight's recovery." I look around my living room, finding that even the parts still alien to me are now made familiar by my mobility aids and assortments of papers, potions and props. I seem to have established my physical self very quickly. I take my sleeping tablet, carry out my well-practised routine and take myself to bed, fearfully and carefully.

14. Home and Where My Heart Is

I've now been home for a whole week. Although it's proving to be an exhausting challenge, I'm certainly trying to prove myself up to it so, apart from one night when I stayed at Sam's after going there for dinner (for company as much as anything else) I have been here the whole time.

So far, the rats and mice that plague my head seem to be staying away for the most part, although I'm still cursed by them even when they're not around for three simple reasons:

1) I expect them to show up, so every movement I spy from the corner of my eye strikes fear.
2) I'm in my own home, on my own street and with my own garden. Real, flesh and blood rats and mice are part of everyday living, so when I potter in the garden I expect them to be there too. Of course, to reassure myself, I can remind myself that they are all well contained in my head but as reassurances go, this isn't one to shout about!
3) My fears are starting to focus, obsessively I know, on the landing window. It's over the kitchen roof and in my mind's eye, the window to my day-mares, it's a convenient entry point for the rats. Much as I'm struggling with the stairs, I have to keep going up and checking that the window's closed. Whilst I'm up there, I also put the toilet seat down, because these rats they are crafty, so very crafty.

#

And so into the last week or so of July. Sam's finished with work for the summer holidays, so I have plenty of extra chances to catch up with her and Evie. Today, we've had coffee together at Sam's house, as our plan is for me to come with her to Evie's library group this afternoon. The trouble is though, that being back home is more exhausting than I thought and any extra outings, including just coming out to Sam's house, seem to take a lot out of me. So, although I say that I might go with her, I get to the point where I realise that I'm just too tired to be able to go. Ok, so I know it's a library and a session of quiet reading and the fun of books with little ones - hardly a noisy environment which will have my senses jangling, but this is just the kind of day where I've already done to much just by coming to Sam's.

I tell her that I'd rather not come to the library and she says that's fine. We agree that I'll get a lift home with her when she goes to the library or at least, that's what I think we agree. Instead, a little while after, she decides not go to the baby group but will instead go for a walk, so she mentions me going home.

"Whenever you are going out" I agree, thinking that sounds fine.

"Well, you can go now if you want to, or in a few minutes," Sam tells me.

So I sit in the living room and to be honest, I just blank out a bit, not thinking of anything much, until Sam suggests again, "I said I can take you now if you want."

"I thought I said whenever you are going out would be ok?" I reply, which is genuinely how I remember the conversation.

Sam now has a face like thunder and the rumble starts. "You're sitting there with your arms crossed like you're waiting for me!"

Again I repeat that I thought we had agreed that whenever she was leaving would be ok.

"Well, I'm feeding the baby now."

My blood starts to run cold, but at the same time begins to boil because it's obvious now that an eruption is brewing between us, I just hadn't expected it. Whatever happens between us, it just triggers something off in both of us.

"All this changing, all these options, it's hard to cope with," I offer, sharing how it feels from my side, a no-blame way out to give us the chance to reach an accord.

"It's bloody hard for me to cope too and I have a 12 month old to look after!" she shouts in response.

Something inside me shuts down. This is too much, what with all the offers to take me home I feel she just wants me to go and, to be honest, it's what I want to do.

"I can get a cab if it's difficult," I tell her, realising as the words tumble out that this may not be as helpful an offer as it had sounded in my head.

Her response is swift "that's your cop out."

She drives me back mostly in silence as, for the moment, there seems little more to say between us. I unlock the front door, slightly more shaky than usual and stumble inside. Oh, how it disturbs me when this happens and it's such a shame, such a change from last week when we had less contact and things were so even, so positive between us. Whatever it is, whether it's the Encephalitis, whether it's the steroids, I don't know what but it's so difficult to cope and things can change in a flash and I can't keep up or I just have to react. I thought at first that she wanted me to be less dependent on her, but when I spill the event out to Frances she says "Sam just wants you more" but just confuses and upsets me more. Is it *this* me she wants, or the old me?

By this evening, I don't know how I've got through the day, feeling so tired and now particularly, so emotional. I reach for the phone and text Sam goodnight, which she returns with the same goodnight kiss. Thinking about what Frances said, in the context of the row, or this "spat" as Sam calls these exchanges which burst out of nowhere, I can see this need, Sam's babyish need to have a proper mother, I can see her as my baby but she's in an adult body; I can't pick her up and kiss it better. As Sam would say "the point I am trying to make is" works the same for me too, I do have a point to make and I just don't seem to be able to say it in a way which can be understood, much less respected. The point *I am trying* to make is that it just causes confusion to have too many options thrown at me, all different and all at the same time. The pressure to make a choice feels enormous and far too overwhelming, particularly when I think I have already made that choice and that a decision has been made. Starting over, in so many ways, is altogether far too much.

#

Today I have my second session with the clinical psychologist, so I tell her about the tiff. I also give her an article on management of Acquired Brain Injury (ABI) from the summer Encephalitis Magazine. In itself, this particular copy epitomises some of what I see as a real impasse in my relationship with Sam. The article discusses the emotional aspects of ABI, including the levels of distress in the patient. Now this, my distress, my crying, is one of the things Sam has found very difficult. Sympathetic to a point but also pragmatic to distraction, she'll ask over and over what's wrong, why are you crying, there must be a reason and on and on and then we'll argue, because she can't understand that sometimes I just cry without knowing why, other than the fact that it must be some sort of release mechanism borne from within the VE or the medication or goodness knows what. The article covered it well, so Frances left the magazine with Sam, not telling me about it until later. To tell the truth, I was a bit annoyed that Frances didn't tell me that she was going to give it to her but of course by then it was done. When I saw the magazine at Sam's the following week I told her I'd like to take it home as I wanted to copy the article for the psychologist.

Sam just said "Ok, I didn't have time to read it."

That really hurt, considering she had said in the past that she does want to help me.

I relay this, through my tears as I pass on the article to the psychologist. She asks me candidly what I thought that was behind the fact she had not read it. I have to think about this. I tell her that at first I thought she's actually not interested, but then I start to think that maybe she does not want to acknowledge that I may be left with ABI. With a surge of realisation, I begin to think that maybe Sam's not as strong as she pretends.

The psychologist then asks me if I think Sam would come to a session. I said I don't know and, as importantly, I don't think I'd know how to ask her. I suggest that maybe, as she has come to many of my other medical appointments, she might be likely to say "I'll think about it" but even as I say this, I know that deep down I'd like a few more sessions on my own first. I need to feel stronger on my own feet before taking that step. The psychologist then moves on, telling me about an adjustment workshop she is holding in December that she thinks will be good for me. I let her put my name down, although I'm mindful of the fact that it might not be necessary by then as the GP has airily impressed on me many times, I "should be feeling better by December."

#

I'm feeling a bit grim. I'm on antibiotics for another urine infection and, having endured the usual pantomime relating to hydro days, have struggled to the hospital pool to be told by the physiotherapist that I'll have to have a "dry" session because she doesn't want me in the pool whilst I'm on antibiotics. Although this cuts out the hassle of the changing room, it's somehow just as exhausting and overwhelming, so instead of gently socialising with the rest of the group, whilst I wait for the transport to take me home, I pull out my journal and start my scribbles. This seems to interest the physiotherapist, who comes over for a chat.

"Do you keep a diary?" she asks.

"Not really," I tell her. "I do write a journal though, you know, every now and again."

We start to talk about writing and I mention that I've been writing a few poems too.

"That's interesting," she remarks but doesn't elaborate, so I then have to ask her why.

She tells me that she does it too, but in a different way. She shares with me that she's doing her doctorate and for her research has interviewed a lot of stroke patients. What she then does is pick the salient bits from the text and converts it to poems.

Part of me isn't quite sure why she's sharing this with me. I mean, in the past we've talked about different people that we have in common as, although I'm not a therapist, my business has meant that I have worked with a lot of occupational therapists and physical therapists over the years. Back in one of those conversations, I told her about one very well known female physical therapist, who's as much a friend as a professional colleague. On that occasion, the hydrotherapist seemed very surprised and, I think, a little bit impressed.

Anyway, as we chat today, and she's sharing snippets about her doctorate, she tells me that she's updating a booklet on special seating and postural control for a charity – the complete remit of my business. She then asks me if I would help her by reviewing her papers, given my background. I'm stunned, speechless. Here, at this very moment in the confines of a therapy session I'm not being seen as a patient, but as the professional person I was before the thief struck. I'm so delighted … this fellow professional sees more in me than just the result of the Encephalitis. Of course I agree readily, not knowing whether it will actually happen or not, but feeling such a boost from the mere fact she's asked me. She also shares that her department is hoping to ask my professional friend to do the same but asks "don't tell her, we haven't contacted her yet." For the first time, in a long, long time, I'm in a conversation which has nothing to do with my hearing and inabilities and everything to do with my old self, I'm back in a professional loop!

#

Ah yes, loops. Pun very much intended there. Less than two days later I'm very much the patient again, rather than the professional because today is the first day of action since Sam's call to Social Services, to ask for assistance for my independent living. As a result, today's action sees a man come to deliver and set up a loop system for my TV.

He seems a very nice man, professional and at pains to make sure I can work the system before leaving me to it. I notice that he's wearing the T-shirt of a National Procurement Company, a company that I, with my business hat on, supply with postural control equipment. There's a strange sense of symmetry coming from this which, if I'm honest, doesn't feel entirely positive in a karmic kind of way, more ironic in a famous last words kind of guise; today I'm finding it very difficult to be on the receiving, rather than the supplying end of assistance.

#

It's almost the end of the month and I'm now gearing myself up for a more frequent return to work, back to business. I'm in today as usual on a Monday, but this one is significant as Lorraine, who has been covering so brilliantly, is dropping back to every other Monday after today, so today's the last day I'll have to familiarise myself with the invoicing and all of the other bits she's been dealing with.

It may not be an easy task. I'm mindful of the fact that I tried on my own last week and just could not get the sequence on the computer right – as I've probably mentioned, I don't find learning new computer skills easy and need lots of practice. So, last week I left a note for her to let her know that I'd need to spend plenty of time on it today, whilst she's here. In the main I'm looking forward to really being back in the swing of things but this part, if I'm honest, I'm really kind of dreading.

When I get there, we exchange our usual cheery greetings and she desk hops to allow me the computer space. This panics me instantly: there's no way I can just get down to it. I feel like I'm already bordering on useless as I have to explain that I need her to talk me through the sequence again, as well as watch me do it and write the steps down for me. I'm flustered and of course listening to her instructions is something of a strain as, despite my hearing aids, she's beside and slightly behind me, rather than in front where I'd be able to see her lips. We complete this process together for one invoice before she moves away again, leaving me her written instructions. I carry on, painstakingly referring to her notes, then back to the computer, mouse, cursor, click, enter, click, check with the notes again. The notes keep blurring up, misty and mischievous as, after four hideously slow invoices, I start to realise that at the speed I'm going I'm likely to be here all day, all week even. I tell Lorraine this and suggest that she might like to take over and get us back on track. She agrees readily enough and I slide away for a moment, unable to quell the tears which have been slowly seeping whilst I've been plodding through those four invoices that I would have completed in 20 minutes flat before January.

#

Even once I'm back home, my morning's work done, I'm feeling sensitive and it's not just because of this morning's hideous awakening to the fact that I'm still very much at the start of my journey to recovery, far less arrived than I had hoped. It's also because a therapist from the sensory team is coming to assess my needs from the hearing aspect. This morning I was at my place of work supplying assistance to the vulnerable, this afternoon, I'm right back there amongst them.

Sam arrives, both for moral support and to be the extra pair of ears needed for if I have to take my aids out for the assessment and such. The therapist arrives shortly after and we have a brief chat of introduction before she starts her appraisal of my situation.

As usual, I find any kind of questions confusing and there are lots of questions. She asks how my walking is and I answer "good" because, to me, it is much improved – there are times, particularly when my ears aren't too bad, my balance is good, I'm not too tired and don't have to far to walk indoors then I can even go without my sticks! So yes, pretty darn good! However, Sam reminds me, and informs the therapist that although it's good in relation to January, actually it's not good in relation to prior-Encephalitis, in relation to the old me. This, of course, sets my tears flowing.

On the whole, we spend about 1 ½ - 2 hours of tears and acknowledgment that I'm not managing being deaf, that I can't "do" this deaf bit on my own. But there is something of a positive outcome, some improvements (albeit basics) are agreed upon: I'm to have a better door bell, flashing fire alarms with a vibrating pad under my pillow and a sensor on the phone. To alert me to any of these during the day, I should carry a small sensor pad, something like a pager, which will make me aware of which device is sounding. It will display a picture of the door or the phone etc so that I know which area needs my attention.

As the session comes to an end, I'm feeling like I'm punch-drunk, like it's all happened to me and around me, much less with me. I'm so glad it's over. As I sit back with a cup of tea afterwards and try to settle my sensibilities I realise that I've found it particularly hard for two reasons. For one thing, it's taken so long because the information about the service and what was involved that we were originally given over the phone has been contradicted completely by the reality of this assessment. But then, as a professional in this kind of industry I should kind of have expected that, as I know many providers with whom that's the case.

And secondly? Ah yes, secondly. It's the emotional factor again, rearing its weeping head because what I've found really hard to cope with is the fact that Sam has once again behaved as she always does at these appointments – she comes and sits beside me and pats me on the back in a kindly sort of way but I want to shriek at her, "why do you only do this at appointments? Is it so that people think you are always like this?" whereas in contrast, when alone together, the reality is that my crying always brings criticism or confrontation. And of course today is no exception. Once the therapist leaves, Sam launches into that very same lecture: "if only you could get over this emotional bit and be more pragmatic about what you need, it would be easier."

I want to shout "because I don't need to be pragmatic about what I need, I know what I need, damn it, what I need is to be able to hear. I want to be *me*, the me I used to be six months ago!" But I don't shout, I'm too tired, far too tired.

The rest of the afternoon's taken up with chores, Sam has offered to help me do a few jobs as my sister's coming and I want to make up her bed as well as change my own. Then Sam offers to run the hoover through, which she does, bless her, on what I think is the hottest day of the year so far. Whilst she's running around in the heat, doing my chores, I look after the baby which I almost find the hardest job of everything I've had to do today. Hot and finding her feet, she's like a slippery little eel, she just keeps on wriggling. And then, suddenly, in a flurry of goodbyes and baby waves, they are gone, home. Barely able to concentrate with fatigue, I throw myself together some sort of dinner, mainly salad, I think and then trudge up the stairs to bed.

It's one of those long, light evenings and I don't have to fear the dark and my nocturnal visitors just yet, so at the moment I am tearful, more than fearful. Once again I'm crying without pause, sobbing once again for all I have lost, for myself and for my daughter – she is just so different now and yet so much her same old self and I am so different now and constantly wishing for my same old self.

#

The month ends on a very tired note, I'd love to feel full and excited about what I've achieved this month: returning back home, being at work ... like this week, for three days out of five. OK, so they weren't full days, but they were full enough for me. Yet all the way through them I've been so exhausted even before I get going each day, like I'm stupid for sleep. Despite that though, I've made the effort to get into the office and do what I can, returning home theoretically before I'm too tired, which is the epitome of appropriately pacing myself. In reality though, I'm always still there when I realise I've overdone it and so then return home in a state of complete fatigue and fuddle. There's another, devastating reality too, which exhausts me just to think about it; you see, I know that what I'm doing, this work which is exhausting me so, it isn't even 'real' work by comparison to what I did before ... now it's more like just putting in the time.

This fuddle itself has lost me vital hours of sanity this week. My bank statement's just come through so I've been checking it avidly; my earlier obsession about my pennies still lingers, despite my progress in other areas. According to the statement I've spent £500 – a big round sum, which should be memorable but isn't. I have no idea what this money was for, where I have spent it. I crash through my piles of papers looking for receipts, scour my bags and pockets for my cheque book to look at the stubs but can't find those either.

Exhausted, frightened and of course very tearful, I phone Sam, explaining every part, including the tiredness and about the £500. I sob that I have no idea about it and I can't find any paperwork to help me get to the bottom of it. Amongst the sobs, I tell her I'm afraid that I've left my cheque book out in a shop or something awful.

"Mum, you haven't lost it" she says, simply. "You've just mislaid it." Then she tells me, as she always does when I cry, that I'm probably just tired, to which I reply, "I know I am, I just told you that." So our warm moment of sharing and help is once again scarred with misunderstanding and some kind of resentment which I can no more put a finger on than I can put a hand to my cheque book.

Which does turn up, of course, along with the confirmation that the £500 payment was to my credit card. Losing things though has the ability to just make me "lose it" in all contexts ... it's a constant, nagging and debilitating worry. I've lost so many things in this house, spent hours looking for things only to find them in the very places where I've been looking. Things seem to disappear and reappear as if by magic and nothing, nobody can convince me that they were there all along. I know they weren't, because I checked!

15. And Breathe Out – A Pause for Therapy

While the NHS are marvellous at keeping people alive, in my experience they do little to keep people living. So, in pursuit of improved health, accelerated progress and a greater sense of doing something to help myself, I've had an ongoing search for therapy to support me with any and all of these, throughout my Encephalitis journey.

Of course this therapy journey has, like my recovery itself, been frustrated by several things, not least:

* The all-consuming urge to get back to Dr. Shen for the assistance I knew would bring me considerable relief. This yearning unfortunately remained unfulfilled for a significant time whilst I was stuck with a body unable to make a journey, along with the need for someone to take me on a regular basis. Unfortunately not everyone is as dedicated, accepting or committed to this as I am, which has exaggerated both my difficulties and my frustrations.
* The fact that NHS therapies which were made available to me were so limited, both in their scope and effects. In the end, I received hydrotherapy and treatment from the clinical psychologist, but little else, despite the ravages of the thief's actions on my body and brain.
* As such, any and all complementary therapies I sought came at a personal financial cost.
* Until I could find out if my private health insurance would cover me (a) for a diagnosis of Encephalitis and (b) for the cost of rehabilitative therapies, I could not afford to 'try' things out. I'm always prepared to dig deep from my own diminishing purse for Dr. Shen's acupuncture and herbs because I've always known how much this benefits me, but I just don't have the means for the "let's try and see ..." exploration and pursuit of other therapies, much as I'm desperate to try anything which presents itself even with the vaguest glimmer of hope for some improvement to my situation.

Yet somehow, over the long period of my recovery, I seem to spend a fortune on various therapies. As such, I think I may have tried most of the therapies out there as I've tried to heal myself, make an effort to improve my situation or get the right therapeutic support to do so. In truth I left almost no stone unturned, so what follows is a list of what I've tried, not what I necessarily endorse or recommend for anyone else. Everyone's Encephalitis or ABI recovery is as individual as they are and responses to therapies will be very much the same. So, with that in mind, my list has included:

- Carnelian stone healing
- Marcasite bracelets and rings
- Acupuncture
- Energy healing
- Feng Shui in my home
- Crystal Healing
- Cawthorn Cooksey ~ a support regime of just two or three sessions, offered through an NHS physiotherapist. This teaches a programme of "kitchen sink" exercises to practice at home, to assist with balance
- Amatsu ~ a hands-on body balancing therapy
- Emotional Freedom Techniques (EFT) ~ also known as 'tapping'
- NHS Hydrotherapy – plus paying for private use of the hydropool
- NHS Clinical Psychology

My earliest therapies in the journey are of course the local acupuncture and massage that I found in the holistic healing centre close to Sam's house. By October 2008, after a few months of visiting her, the therapist mentions Emotional Freedom Techniques to me. I have some recollection of this, from a Reiki therapist I used to go to. At that time, she had demonstrated EFT to me but I'd told her that I didn't think it was for me. This time, my acupuncturist offers to book a session in, to go through it with me. However, I still really don't think it will offer any benefits, so again I reject the offer.

Theoretically of course, EFT offers plenty that interests me, from therapeutic and physical angles, as well as from the perspective of the very emotionally traumatised situation I now find myself in. As a therapy, Emotional

Freedom Techniques (EFT) are based on meridian energy therapy, like acupuncture, except EFT involves tapping into the source of our bodies' hidden wounds, in order to uncover, acknowledge and enable healing, free from negative emotions and energies. It's also supposed to relate closely to the effectiveness of talking therapies as verbalisation is part of the process, which I'm sure would benefit me but at the moment and when considering my experience with the Reiki therapist, alongside the healing relationship from this acupuncturist, I don't feel that EFT would offer me anything else. I tell her that I'll think about it but, in my heart of hearts, I'm not that optimistic that it's the right kind of therapy for me, especially at the £35 an hour my acupuncturist charges!

However, when I get home a letter awaits me; an invitation to join in another of the training days for counsellors, a way of maintaining continued professional development. It seems really important to me to try to attend, whatever the topic, so that I can get practising again but as I painstakingly read through the invitation, it seems that the theme for the day is EFT and instantly I'm reminded of an old saying, that when you need to learn something the teacher finds you.

#

It's approximately a month later when I attend the workshop. It's being facilitated by Ranjana Appoo, a fascinating lady of Indian heritage. Beautiful from within and so pleasant, so light in spirit and obviously extremely passionate about her subject, her experience and knowledge make it an absorbing day and we strike up an immediate rapport.

But however interesting the topic, as usual, my hearing difficulties make it extremely difficult for me to engage with everything, so I miss a lot of what is said. I'm able to fill some of the gaps with the literature she provides us with. EFT works like acupuncture without needles, tapping the points and including verbalisations and affirmations affecting a psychological shift, depending on what you are targeting.

The day is delivered in sections – therapy theory and practice. It seems so much more intuitive and purposeful than when I experienced it last year … I just wasn't impressed with it then. When the time comes that Ranjana requests a volunteer for the practical demonstrations, I don't hesitate and she readily engages with me, demonstrating the tapping treatment using my ramshackle body, whilst everyone follows, concentrating on the same patterns. I come away entirely impressed and convinced that my previous negative experience of it was to do with its delivery; this lady's energy is palpable and the experience all-encompassing. I have plenty now to think about and my first plan of action is, before the day is even over, to make an appointment with her for a private session.

#

I can't believe that, having decided to turn down EFT from two practitioners I have now found a practitioner who is delivering what appears to be something of a life-saving therapy to me. It takes no time to get started as Ranjana books to see me at her centre which is, thankfully, accessible to me. Although she is choosy about who she works with, she clearly remembers me from the workshop and wants to work with me. Just from our involvement in the short demo sessions, she can feel the work that needs to be done, the healing that I both need and crave.

We start off with weekly sessions where, just like with the clinical psychologist, I cry, mostly throughout. Ranjana is kind and non-judgemental and of course emotions fit right into Emotional Freedom Therapy! So I bring along those emotions, with such openness that the tissues are already on standby for when I arrive. I feel embraced by her understanding and within a few sessions start to feel a shift in my own understanding of what's happened to me and how to manage myself, the outcome of it all.

Another shift occurs, but for Ranjana too. Her usual way of working is to offer two to six sessions only, with a focus on teaching traditional EFT methods to offer a support structure and empowerment. EFT is not supposed to be a long term, therapist-led intervention but instead provides clients with self-help tools to continue the work. Yet my healing needs are so much wider than this. Ranjana's own personal experiences draw her to want to help in my case, over and above her usual routines, to help resolve some of the emotional effects of the thief, or at least empower me to manage how I feel about these hideous, lasting effects. Ranjana's grandmother in India had Encephalitis and lost her own senses – sight as well as hearing, so her empathy for my situation is genuine and well embedded in experience of what it's like to be catapulted overnight into this situation, so helpless, so disabled and so very lost.

Ranjana offers her special rate for me, to help accommodate more long-term EFT treatment. For the first year I see her weekly and we concentrate on traditional EFT to help address and then start to heal some of my pressing issues.

It's hard to explain the effects of EFT. As someone who has experienced acupuncture and has a background in counselling, with transactional analysis as my model of choice, I'd been finding, since the thief, that my background, qualifications and training didn't count for much anymore. Those were attributes of the woman I used to be, not she who sits in this chair now.

Yet EFT literally taps into what I know and have experienced, even some of those aspects that I'd believed to be lost, and I feel like I bring something of myself, of my own, to the sessions. Not just the tears and the problems, but the solutions too ... the sense of empowerment arising from the EFT is considerable and something that I want to continue to explore, to maintain my healing as well as develop my own understanding. In order to do this I have to be able to acknowledge all my losses, physical and emotional, a tall order for someone who's struggling with acceptance even at a basic level.

#

It really isn't easy. One of the other aspects that I had not foreseen is that the thief also seems to have stripped away the benefits of any direct counselling I've had in the past, so by the time I start EFT, it's like I have to work through all of those old issues again, issues which pre-date the Encephalitis yet have resurfaced for old times' sake. This makes no sense to me. When I think about how emotional I am and the issues and situations which rouse such anger, anxiety and sadness in me, issues which I think to myself I should be handling better because I've already put them to bed; I should be 'over it', it's dealt with. Eventually I start to realise that I'm not being useless by falling prey to those feelings all over again; yes, I put them to bed, but the thief woke them back up. So now I have to look to the EFT to connect with that deeper layer, like peeling away the layers of an onion and of course the deeper we cut it, the more it makes us cry! And cry I do.

#

My EFT sessions develop quickly into varying routines. At the start of sessions, Ranjana 'reads' me quickly to help decide the pace and depth of the session. So at each session she decides whether it should be a gentle session or a deeper session (sometimes the deeper stuff just pours out anyway). She takes my pulse, just as Dr. Shen does at the start and says the pulse doesn't lie, that my appearance is stronger than my body and the pulse tells her what is needed. As a result, we work on things that have upset or bothered me over the weekend, the vulnerability of travelling, the lack of connection with what is going on, having to constantly ask and feeling like a small, helpless child.

Sometimes these issues are drawn out of me, I don't know I need to work on them until I'm there, but at other times I arrive with one of my lists, my to-do list of the things I'm anxious to deal with: the fear; the babysitting; selling the business.

My poem, The Woman I Used to Be becomes a feature of the sessions. Having told Ranjana about this poem, it's now here with us and my job is to try to read it through, so that we can try to break through my tears. Of course, to start with I never get far with the reading of the poem and the tears are indeed painful, it feels, more than cleansing. I cry buckets whilst Ranjana taps away the tears of trauma, to allow instead healing tears to come through, to do their work and wash away the illness.

During one of these poem sessions, I'm more traumatised than usual, because tomorrow is the anniversary of the hospitalization; she says my birthday for starting a new life, starting anew. I try to hold this to me as an empowering thought, for the me I am now, but to be honest it doesn't bring me much power, at least initially. That comes later. Much later.

#

As with all aspects of my recovery, my progress is slow. Sometimes, when I am particularly low, stressed, anxious and my head is relentlessly noisy, I think, dear Lord will this head ever be quiet? Will I ever be able to think clearly, what I want to think, without these distorted thoughts, these violent, disturbing thoughts? And then there are the rats, always the rats. I add all of this onto my list to work on with Ranjana the next day.

When I'm there, I'm always astounded by the issues that surface in the tapping process. Today is no different. I take my fears around Evie and my fear of the rats, both fears that continue to reoccur, day and night, no peace, no reprieve.

The thing is that EFT can literally tap into all aspects of the brain, even deep seated memories and traumas. Aspects of my current fears, which I associate with the Encephalitis are those bad memories which actually pre-date the illness but were literally unlocked by the thief. As such, it's easy to identify where the rats are coming from. They're from my childhood, from my parents' fear of dirt. Wiel's disease, which was a real threat on a farm, but not only this threat of disease, also for our food, our root crops and grain store, their invasion of our space. As children we were always told to be careful about hand washing and the exaggerated fear of this invasion is a common theme of my own hallucinations and nightmares. The fear of this is dealt with fairly quickly in this session, but we do come back to it, time and again, over many more.

My fears around Evie are similarly deep-seated and my ability, or lack of it, to protect her takes a little more time, or should I say much more time is spent on this.

The main purpose of the EFT, throughout this first year is to move my poor, sore brain and battered emotions on from these disturbing memories. Each session sees another trauma released which never comes back in the same way. There's an element of re-living each episode which is an awful but necessary as part of the journey. But it's not just my journey, it's the journey of the trauma, moving it from the past, into the present and then out of the door, gone, so that I can move on from being trapped in those moments, those hideous, exaggerated memories, and then start to heal.

Of course it's complicated, with many of these disturbing thoughts and memories released by the thief but originating elsewhere. However, the tapping and exploring enables us to move across time, to use all my remaining senses to investigate the best ways to identify and release the emotion, heal the pain. This too fits in with the fact that Encephalitis seems to have taken me to a pre-stage, with only an infantile capacity for managing how I feel, which the EFT also taps into and challenges. This makes it a very intense process, but it's so useful for me just now.

And it's not just what it achieves. Part of the reason I find EFT so effective is that, like visits to the clinical psychologist, it's a place where I can safely have a release of emotions which I don't have to explain or justify, those emotions that it's not safe to reveal anywhere else.

#

Just like the way my ABI has in turn affected my entire physical self, so the EFT aims to treat the whole body through the head. Elements are revisited to help target the different areas, the aches, the pains, the intemperate limbs, the headaches and the incontinence. It's no cure-all, I know that, but there's a benefit to all because all my physical and emotional symptoms are of course so intricately entwined. The big break-through though, in the first six months of EFT is that I am able to acknowledge my anger at my losses. Of course I always kind of knew I was angry, to tell the truth, even after all this therapy I'm still pretty bloody angry about it a lot of the time, but I needed Ranjana, as it turns out, and the EFT, to channel me to be able to acknowledge it, to deal with it and to gain benefit from Energy Psychology, instead of allowing the anger to remain as another source of the thief's poison coursing through my body.

#

By the second year, I'm visiting Ranjana for three-weekly sessions in each month. Much of this therapy now centres on my own discovery about who I was and who I am now. A shift, subtle but gradual, creeps into my subconscious. Our focus is not about returning me to who I was but to find out who I am now and to mould me into that same kind of self-responsible, resourceful woman, a role model for others. It's incredible that Ranjana can rally in me this echo of the woman I was and I find this part of my old self, part that wasn't lost at all. Ranjana facilitates this link for me and helps me to build my new foundation the right way. All this time, I've been assailing the medical profession and berating myself for my lack of independence, but now realise that what I can have instead is a different thing: freedom ~ of thoughts, spirit, heart and emotion. None of this "think positive, you'll soon be back to normal" mantra; forcing a positivity is never going to bring back my independence, but allowing this freedom to face up to and deal with those negatives does itself bring positive elements. I start to develop my own inner force, that inner faith which I quickly learned to trust whilst all the time my faith in my God and other people was sorely tested. It surprises me, yet at the same time it doesn't, that I was right to have faith in myself all along, that I knew I was right: to thine own self be true, as they say.

It helps too that Ranjana creates such good energy and is such a pleasant person to be with. She not only treats me as a person, she also has me in her professional mind too and does things like asking her professional colleagues for suggestions on other ways of working with me, of helping me to heal. To her this is no big deal, just a kindness, although any little kindness still seems to be a pretty big deal for me. From time to time she returns to India and when she comes back she brings gifts: earrings, pain lotion, a tissue box cover and a calendar, more of her generous spirit shining through.

#

That's not to say I don't still have my dark days. One of these days I arrive for my session and remark about how angry the sea looks today.

"Are you?" Ranjana asks me, looking me directly in the eyes. She's right of course, I'm projecting it, the sea represents my anger. I tell her I just want to be dead, because that's how low I am feeling.

She doesn't judge me for saying such a shocking thing, even after her own grandmother's perseverance in the face of even greater adversity. If anything, she is more understanding of why I feel it, say it. That's the thing with working with a holistic healer, they will understand that what you say is a reflection of more than one actual event, one physical or emotional loss. Despite what I've just declared, these sessions, this non-judgemental support has been a life saver for me.

I think this is all part of it, for those like me, afflicted with some terrifying illness which leaves such devastating effects. Recovery seems like such a huge thing and with the NHS offering so little support for the sum of those wrecked parts, the whole person afflicted, that therapy, whatever therapy most suits the individual, should really be some kind of option. This is an incredibly tough journey and although sometimes I think that I am going nowhere fast, there's real joy and satisfaction in receiving the right therapeutic support – to be able to cry, be upset, be sad, be anything that comes up and not to have to explain why, just accept and be accepted, not being told to think positive or, worse, that I am wallowing in this but instead being respected for who and how I am. That in itself promotes healing of a kind.

For me, EFT with Ranjana, acupuncture and herbs with Dr. Shen as well as, to some extent, the time with the clinical psychologist, have been the things which have worked for me. It might not suit everyone and there's a whole raft of genuine therapies as well as snake-oil salesmen out there to sift through, but finding the right therapy seems to me to be an absolute essential to stand any chance of recovering yourself after Encephalitis.

#

By the latter part of my second year of treatment, I start to attend workshops, to find out more about the process and to begin training as an EFT practitioner. I try to bring some of my other counselling and psychology knowledge in to apply it, but of course I have forgotten so much. I do still have some of my intuition though, which helps and I'm surprised not only how much benefit I'm getting from the treatment itself but also from practising, so this too becomes part of my journey: from seeking healing, to self-healing and then becoming an EFT practitioner myself. If I step to the outside and look in, at my old Encephalitis-riddled self, I still can't see that it's been possible, surely it's too much to expect from recovery, a step too far? But no, small steps have made it possible, small steps very much in the right emotional and physical direction.

We move into including Jin Shin Jyutsu, an ancient hands-on healing, as part of my EFT sessions, a movement away from traditional EFT. For some time recently we've also been practising a process Ranjana is developing, called Liberating Touch. After she attends a course and speaks with the tutor about my particular problems, especially my stress and anxiety with the raging tinnitus, Ranjana suggests that our sessions should take on a more intensive focus, so for the third year we move into a pattern where I see her for an hour a day, five days a week and then have a much longer break between appointments. We start this in the May, and when we book it I'm a little anxious, concerned that it will be tedious and hard work, what with fitting in all the appointments for everything else going on. In the practice though, it turns out to be an absolute gift, to get all this treatment in a week. I feel blessed and, what's more, I do feel the benefit.

#

Over my time with Ranjana, both she and I gradually see the improvements. Sometimes I'll see her and think that I don't have much to say or deal with. On one such occasion I started to chit-chat instead, telling her about my Uncle's deterioration in health and the fact he's in hospital post-stroke. All of a sudden I'm back in hospital myself and to all intents and purpose dead. This, out of nowhere, becomes the first time I've had to deal with this experience and I'm so glad it shows up here, with someone I can trust to take me through it. From feeling I had nothing to say, we end up with a major therapeutic session focusing on and around my death, on my not knowing if I was dead or alive. And of course my continuing belief that a big part of the real me actually died from the Encephalitis.

#

One thing which is interesting for me in my journey towards healing is that my main method of outpouring, my journaling and notes, dries up on those days I am focused on EFT. I find I don't want to write it all down, it's like I have enough to do, to face up to when I'm there, it's so intense and I don't want to over-analyse it with a second, scribbled outpouring. My words are already out there and I just want to let them be.

#

I continue with EFT, both through my sessions with Ranjana, my attendance at workshops and my progress as a level 3 practitioner. Whilst it's also helped with my healing, it has restored my self-confidence in a way which is wider, better than anything else I have tried since I have been affected by Viral Encephalitis. It has helped me to reclaim my faith, in some form, certainly restoring my faith in myself. Now, at this time of bringing together the good, the bad and the so very ugly of my Encephalitis journey, I continue to work on acceptance and expectation.

Personal note

My explorations of these therapies are part of my own story, my own journey. I don't recommend any particular therapy, as the 'right' one for others as such things can only be 'right' on an individual basis ... one man's meat and all that.

However, what I will say is that sometimes therapy, any therapy, which involves one to one time with a therapist can be beneficial because it offers safe, undivided attention, which on that rough road to recovery, we could all do with at times ~ for ourselves and as a break for those supporting us. For me, the best way of describing the benefits I've experienced from Emotional Freedom Techniques as part of my rehabilitation are not words from my own journals, but from the eloquent George Bernard Shaw:

"Life isn't about finding yourself. Life is about creating yourself."

Certainly EFT is helping me to create, and accept, the person I am and the life I now have.

16. A Cloudy Summer

August 2008. A month of fun and sun traditionally, although I'm not sure fun will feature much this year! Still, I live in hope, if not of the fun then at least the sunshine, as I drag myself out of bed, away from the night monsters and into each new day.

I'm going up to London today, to Sutton to see Dr Shen. Sam's supposed to be coming around 9ish as she's taking me, to enjoy a day out too. So, I'm surprised to see her coming through the front door at 8.30, in desperate need of a shower. It turns out they've got a leak in the bathroom at home and have had to turn the water off. Although a distraction and, for me, an aberration to our plans which might normally have me flustered, it's all fine, almost in a fun way, like the old days of having her home as a teenager. OK, so that was a different time, different house, different life, but to see her flitting about swathed in towels, trailing steam, scent and splashes behind her as I plod along with my chores, is comforting. I feel a sense of homeliness and happiness that I think has been missing for quite a while although I didn't know it, didn't realise it until just now.

So, we're both in a good mood as we set off to Sutton. After last month's long trip to Dorset, I find this journey quite manageable, although I'm a little achy, but the roads are good and we arrive in plenty of time to even grab a bit of lunch before my appointment. Again, it's pleasant, cheerful, I'm really starting to feel like I'm on a day out with my daughter, as much as a trip to see my herbalist.

Speaking of which, the appointment is a good one too. I produce my list (which of course I have been preparing solicitously for weeks now), the catalogue of symptoms the thief and the ensuing medication have left behind: my headaches; prominent veins; continued incontinence; storming tinnitus; body still swollen but slowly deflating; skin on ankles and elbows sore. She takes it all in, studiously and then offers me acupuncture. Of course, I seize the chance so it's up onto the table where she confidently and precisely applies her needles: back first, then front. Those needles hit the spot every time and the relief is enormous.

I say to her "I'm glad this is a treatment and not a torture" but actually I know that even if it did feel grim and awful, I'd probably still come willingly because it helps so much. I leave her on a high note, clutching more virus tea, raw herbs for 3 weeks and an appointment for the same time in two weeks, which will go straight onto my calendar as a lifeline in my personal timeline.

Sam drives us back home and it's so calm, so genial, it's starting to feel to me like August is already a turning point. We chat and have the odd laugh: we're more than just civil, really companionable. I feel that I can really mark this one down as a good day, a very good day.

We go back to Sam's for a cup of tea, then leave Evie with her dad so that we can finish off our day with a trip to the supermarket for the weekend shop. I feel so proud of myself, getting through all of these things and of Sam for making it such as pleasant time. Even the trail around the supermarket feels more like an outing and less like a chore, especially as I'm buying treats to share with Frances, who arrives for another short visit tomorrow.

Sam drops me home with my shopping, helping me in with the bags, still chatting about one of her friends. I say something, I can't remember what, my usual comment before thinking but I'm sure it was innocent enough – certainly innocently meant. I watch her face change and the shutters come down. She heaves the last carrier bag onto the kitchen counter and turns to leave, but before she goes she says "I just want to clarify."

I'm not sure what she means but I quickly point out that I was just making a comment, the whole issue makes no difference to me. I also point out that her own views she has made about the person have also been differing, so it's confusing for me.

Her face doesn't change. "As I said earlier, we are allowed to change," she says. Her words hang in the air long after she leaves and I cry, for a lovely day gone sour, for the fact that apparently change is allowed except, it seems, for me.

#

Frances has arrived, hale and hearty. We share simple dinners, the "clean" diet I have been craving and trying to follow suits her. We eat trout, salad and new potatoes and have plenty of chats but also factor in some earlier nights than during our last visit together: it's not just me who's feeling tired this time around!

On her last day we visit Sam, who's arranged a family barbeque. Unfortunately Simon's in bed, unwell. He's been struggling with a bad cold and fever for the past week or so and it seems to have returned, so quite rightly he's staying out of our way and nursing it, as they're meant to be going on holiday next week. The weather's cloudy though and altogether a bit grim, so Sam cooks indoors for us and we all make the best of it. It's grand to be together, apart from poor old Simon, and Evie keeps us all entertained with her little ways.

By 6.30 we're back home, to give Sam a chance for a quiet time settling Evie to bed and to give Frances the chance to finish packing for tomorrow. As I settle into my armchair, I don't feel quite right. My stomach is dancing and I just want to close my eyes. I have that watery, vomit sensation but I really don't want to vomit, it has far too many associated memories for me: I don't want to be sick, I mustn't be sick.

An early night seems to be in order for both of us. Frances comes to check on me as I settle, wearily, queasily into my bed. For some reason, the urge to vomit is now beaten by the involuntary need to cry. I'm lying in my bed sobbing, really wailing, streams of tears and snot as a tide of all the old fears come flooding back, I'm tortured and terrified. Poor Frances holds my hand as my fears flood out.

"I don't want to die!" I cry, before wailing more about my other fears: my children's safety; their driving; their travelling; their health; was the sickness going to start all over again; more hospital looming; hideous hallucinations just waiting to creep in … where does this stop? And it so it doesn't, I can only let the tide take me, whilst my sister gently lies on the bed beside me, to keep me afloat.

#

Another Saturday has come around with it another trip to London to see Dr. Shen. Sam's volunteered to drive me again and she's here so that we can set out for 10.30, which gives us plenty of time like before, to arrive before the baby needs a bottle and so that we can have a bit of lunch before my treatment, which usually lasts about an hour and fifteen minutes.

The doctor seems as pleased to see me as I am to see her, greeting me warmly as usual. I'm so pleased that one of the first things she says to me is that my moon face has gone. Now I don't usually like to be anywhere around the words "moon face" but in this case I'm more than happy to make an exception. She says that all the puffiness is gone and that I seem to have made a lot of progress since my last visit.

We both agree that the herbs I'm on really do seem to be doing me good, so she provides me with more. She also gives me the good news that I can stop drinking the virus tea, once I've finished the sachets I still have. Yes, this is good news, but also a little scary, like another little prop being removed because what I don't really want, more than almost anything apart from my family to be safe, is for the virus to come back.

The acupuncture treatment eases my symptoms and my fears though, and I relax thoroughly throughout the process. I do so love coming here, seeing the doctor and knowing that I'm going to be feeling the benefits from her acupuncture almost instantly. However, it's an exhausting four hour round trip – and that's just for me, the passenger, it's also a lot to ask of Sam although she offers most of the time and says that she doesn't mind the outing.

We're a little quieter today, on the way home. I know I'm exhausted and I'm sure she is too, with Evie to look after all day as well. I'm hoping she's not dwelling on last time we made this trip, as I too am also trying not to do. I have no reason to expect anything other than for today to be totally positive and, thanks to Sam's kindness in bringing me and Dr. Shen's enthusiasm for my improvement (and my face), it really does feel like a good day.

After Sam drops me home, I settle with the feel good vibe, making myself a light supper, trying to do a crossword and then dragging myself wearily up to bed. I'm exhausted, my whole body feels like I just can't ask it to do another thing but, thanks to the acupuncture, when I do finally fall into bed there's already some relief from the leg and muscle pains. Yes, this has been a good day.

#

Of course, my days are still very much a mixture of good and bad but after all this time I've finally made the connection that a considerable number of what I'd call bad days are also those where Sam and I have a tiff, words, disagreement, misunderstanding ... whatever the hell you'd want to call what seems to happen between us. There's almost certainly some kind of chicken-egg situation going on, some deep psychology at work that comes from the fact that we're both a victim of my circumstances since the thief struck, but I get too tired to work out the reasons for the problems, my energy's better spent trying to find ways to fix it. Mostly, I think, short bursts of time together seem fine, so I'm making the decision to keep a little distance between us and not to ask for too much help. Instead I shall stay away a bit and concentrate on short, positive visits as the best way forwards.

As well as trying to even out our relationship, I'm trying desperately to be independent, so I try not to ask her to do anything for me, apart from the odd practical bits which are OK when she's here, like carrying something up stairs or lifting something for me. I can manage better this way really and I'm really trying hard, or as much as my memory allows me at least, to not get involved in any conversation or discussion with her on topics which could raise issues. For myself, this feels like a significant move, not necessarily in the action I'm taking, but the fact that I feel strong enough emotionally to do this. I guess it's a true sign that I'm a bit stronger now. I really feel, after all these long months, that I can manage this, whereas there's no way I had the strength before.

Of course, I'm not ignoring them, my own flesh and blood, especially not after all they've done to help me. I'd really just like to be useful back and not just burdensome or troublesome. With this in mind, because Sam, Simon and Evie are going to France on Wednesday, I've offered to help out today, Monday, perhaps with a bit of packing. So here I am. I do a little ironing and then read to Evie. I'm just so glad she's too tiny to read for herself and doesn't realise that these early-readers are a real challenge for me in getting used to reading aloud, with speed, expression and understanding. I'm literally going to have to be a page ahead of her when she starts reading for herself!

I then help with a bit more packing, sitting on the bed passing things to Sam, the tried and tested method of take that, leave that kind of packing. It's all going OK but somehow, I feel it creeping in again, the sadness, to do with these bedrooms and suitcases, I think. It just reminds me of how sick and miserable I was whilst I was here, although it's not to do with being at Sam's really. Deep down, I think it could have been said of anywhere I might have been at that point, just that reminder of how sick I've been. Sam invites me to stay for dinner, but she has plenty of other things to do and I really want to keep going with my plan for the short, but sweet times together, so I do, regretfully, decline.

#

It's Tuesday, a work day for me at the office. It's going OK, but under my own steam, my own unsteady pace, or is that gait, really? Sam's insisted on coming in too, to help, even though I tell her that she really doesn't need to, after all Antony will be here tomorrow. Still, as we're both here, we both get on a bit, then she goes ahead to the supermarket and I join her there when I'm ready.

Although we're both in a reasonable humour, I'm starting to notice that she seems to torture herself with decisions like me, I suppose, at my dithering best. Recently we've had days of her really not knowing what to get Simon for his birthday, then she decided but couldn't find what she wanted and it's clearly playing on her mind today. She ponders her options and finally, having made another decision, all she needs to do is go into the shop and pick it up.

"Go," I say, "just go get it ... I'll sit with baby in the car and it will take you two minutes."

I'm trying to be helpful but the response is "I'm not doing it now I'll do it later."

I find it exhausting, all this changing and thinking out loud, so tiring and wearing, like the stress of my own dithering decision making – it's bad enough doing it myself, let alone listening to someone else doing it!

#

I guess it's all part of the stress and the tiredness that I'm in the continuing throes of aches and pains; some days there's not a part of me that doesn't hurt. I'm getting used to two or three days of headaches at a time but I'm trying to stay away from paracetamol and up my water intake instead. To some extent this seems to work and in the last two weeks, between visits to herbalist, I had two days of headaches and no painkillers, which I'm secretly pretty chuffed with myself about … I would so like to be off all these medications, not just because it would be a real sign of having recovered, but because it gets to the point where I don't know if my symptoms are my condition or the side-effects from the medications!

#

I have realised one big source of my underlying stress and it has nothing to do with family or medication, but everything to do with work. The fact is one which I've put off facing for quite a while: I'm not the woman I was. Neither in that very feminine sense of the word, nor the business sense. Yes, I've been ignoring the fact that, actually, the business is too much for me. There's no way I can keep putting upon others to help me run it, I have no business partner to bear the load or buy me out, so I have to sell the business.

At times I'm fairly OK with this decision: it's time to let it go. At other times, I'm very much not OK with it, my business is the last vestige of the professional person I was – to sell it is to acknowledge that person is gone, very much gone.

To be sure though, as much as I can be emotional about the situation, I can also be very practical. So wheels have been set in motion and, although the business has been valued for less than I hoped, I've made the decision to sell. Through my own professional network I've found two interested parties who I intend to approach before I decide to give it to the Transfer Agent, as it would cost a lot less to sell direct. See, head very much managing the heart on this one, although the truth is my head is bearing the brunt of the very real pain of this decision.

17. Keeping up Appearances

I've discovered that Thursday is my worst night's sleep of the week. On Friday morning I take one Androlic Acid, which has to be taken 30 - 60 mins before food with lots of liquid. Then, I have to sit up straight for 30 mins. This is supposed to be the routine, however today I have wakened and taken it at 2am, not realising how out of touch with time I am. For some reason I always need to visit the toilet more on Thursday nights and with my sleep so broken, my nightly fears remain vivid and I take longer to get back to sleep. After such a hard night and with the malarkey which goes along with taking the androlic acid, I read for a while, then I take my breakfast and rest of my medication and read some more. When it comes to getting up for the day, I've been awake for hours and so of course find it hard to get up.

While I carry on with all these activities it gives the impression that I am ok and doing well, which of course I am, if I compare myself to January. We are now in August, a whole seven months on and yes, I'll concede, the improvement since then is significant.

However, if I compare myself to this time last year there is no comparison at all and I cry easily at the thought of it. Last August I was fit and healthy, running up and down to my daughter with her new baby and helping any way I could. I had not long returned from my yoga holiday in Turkey with my sister and had started to make my customarily early Christmas preparations.

Fast forward to now. Now I feel like a pregnant duck, waddling about with what feels like webbed/flat feet and that's when I'm up and about. The effect of gravity also plays its part on the bloody incontinence which just continues, relentlessly. The days that I'm doubly incontinent are just the pits; that constant feeling of not being clean and I'm so afraid of smelling. Thankfully though, despite the tricks of some of my other senses, I've retained a good sense of smell so I'm soon aware if there's a problem there. That said though, by the time I'm able to smell it is usually too late, far too late in polite society. So of course there's never time to relax about such things, I'm always checking and changing.

And moving about less is no answer. Sitting just adds to the stiffness and body pain, basically it's so uncomfortable to walk or sit so whatever position I'm in, I'm distracted by how uncomfortable I am. I find it hard to concentrate on what is being said to me, even on a good day when my ears and hearing aids are working politely together, with less interference or wailing tinnitus. So I appear not to be listening or interested, but have to ask whoever I'm with to pass on their information as just one thing at a time please! All this and acquaintances say "oh I'm glad you're better!" I'm glad too, but it's a comparative better: what people see on the outside doesn't match what I feel on the inside. And I do feel it, on the inside.

Not having a support group makes all these things more difficult. There's no-one to tell you how it was for them or how they coped. My physiotherapist knows of one other lady, just like me a victim to this horrible disease, but over 15 years ago in her case. Having checked with her, my physio gave me this lady's number but of course I mislaid it amongst my precious piles of careful filing, so today she gives it to me again. I resolve to contact her as she lives fairly locally, maybe five or six miles away. I would love to set up some group for people who just want to talk, not go to bowls or such activities that are offered by the ABI group, the only vaguely related support group which is in existence in my area. I would consider going to one of their meetings, but their letters announcing their meetings always arrive after the date of the said meeting, which is almost funny in its alarming messing-with-your-head kind of way!

So, the closest I get to the professional emotional support I need from the NHS is the clinical psychologist. Today she's been running late, so I'm waiting in chairs for what seems like an age, before finally getting in to see her around 1.15. However, I get a whole hour with her, which to be honest I really feel like I need after a break of four whole weeks. A month seems too long really, it leaves me feeling as if I'm coping on my own again. It's good to see her though, although she doesn't seem to make any suggestions for managing or give any guidelines, which an official support group would be able to do, I think. Instead, we seem to have a whole hour of me talking (and yes, still crying) about the damage that this condition has done to me and subsequently to my relationship with my daughter. I'm still just not the me I used to be. And the crying, the endless crying I do whilst I'm here.

Towards the end of the session, she talks again about her group in December called Adjusting to Change. As usual, I tell her that it's my intention to get back to full health by then and of course there's a very professional pause before she reminds me that my progress might be slower or that by December I may have reached a plateau in my recovery. She spells out to me the fact that I have tried to ignore for myself yet conversely tried to get others to recognise and show empathy for: that I've had a huge assault to my brain. She suggests that whatever stage I'm at, I'd find on-going support over this period of adjustment useful. I remind her that I don't really want to adjust to change, I want to get back to being me.

#

Another day, another intervention. Today it's hydrotherapy so the transport duly rolls up at 1.30 and I finally decamp from the window to join them. I say hello to the others on the bus but get little response - some weeks people speak and some they don't. I know that feeling so I leave them to it.

Once there, I wait for my turn, get ready, still painfully slow, then have a shower and get into the pool. The therapist has mild tinnitus in one ear and has been referred to the ENT (Ear, Nose and Throat Department). She tells me that she is being sent for scans and says casually that she's "sure of course you had all that." Of course the truth is rather different, my investigations and appointments take forever and a completely different form, so I tell her "no, I had no nothing like that for my ears."

She does some checks and says my legs are still weak. I ask what she would suggest and she says quickly "more hydro, you are entitled to six sessions." I still have three to take, what with my antibiotics and her absence it has gone on a bit. She asks if I want to do a few more sessions, stay on a bit longer or come twice a week. The choices seem overwhelming to consider back-to-back so I take them one at a time – a few more sessions, well yes, that's what I'm entitled to; stay on a bit longer, probably not, the whole thing is exhausting enough with its current timings; twice a week then? This would seem to be the most beneficial way to really build on progress and I tell her this. She says she would certainly agree but unfortunately she has a long waiting list.

I'm getting a little tired now of this back and forth, of these options which aren't really options. I remind her that I was on the waiting list for the eight weeks I was in hospital and then waited a month when I came out before she saw me.

Rather sheepishly she says "I did not know about you." It turns out that the physical therapist who saw me the day before discharge forgot to put me on the waiting list hence the excessive delay, none of which helps my stiff, stuck body.

As an alternative, she suggests that I could come in the evening but would have to pay. Hmmm, I'm trying to remind myself that I have a professional persona under here and I try to tap into that person, just for a moment, before I say something regrettable. Thankfully, graciously, I point out that I object to this as, other than 3 sessions of hydro, I'm not getting any continuing physical treatment, so I'll come in the day, whenever she can fit me in. She does have a few other suggestions for "in the meantime", including getting a static bike or doing Nordic Walking, apparently there is a class which runs, or rather walks, on the sea front. She says she will get me the info but of course these too are extras with a cost attached to them and I'm about to become unemployed.

#

Another thing, despite those outward appearances of being much improved, I still clutch the shopping list when I go out. To save me walking miles back and forth on myself, the list is now in the order of the shops. For the most part, this is one of my most productive self-help schemes, but it does fall flat on its face when:

* I have company and have to stray from the list because the other person needs to go here or there.

* I have company as I kind of hand over some of my responsibility for myself. I tell them, I need to go here or there – I think there is a confidence in someone else knowing, but it means I absolve myself of a little of my own carefully regained independence and responsibility.

* The supermarket moves everything around, again. It's not until you need things to stay in the same place that you start to notice how frequently they chop and change things about!

#

My son Simon comes to stay for a few days, a mini-break to catch up a bit. It's lovely to have him here and to feel that we're home together, unlike last time, when it felt like we were in a cold, impersonal hotel, somewhere I felt no link to. This place definitely feels like it's my home now.

We spend some gentle days, catching up with each other, spending time with Sam and the baby, going for outings, like summer days out when they were children and we couldn't afford to go on proper days out, just trips here and there.

We get back from one of these outings and I find I've lost my marcasite ring. I know, at least as much as I know anything for sure, that I was wearing it. It must have happened when I was out, maybe in the public loos when I washed my hands? Perhaps it was the soap, maybe it just slipped off? My finger feels bare and unfamiliar without it. Simon helps me to look around the house, just in case, but I'm sure it must have been lost outside and I'm furious with myself for my carelessness.

It hasn't turned up yet and Simon's due to go home. His flight's this evening, so he comes to work with me for the morning. In all, it's not the best morning in the office: the heavy duty stapler breaks, just like that, leaving us unable to do the packing for dispatch. Antony's working today, thankfully, so he pops me up to the stationery suppliers in search of a replacement, but our search is fruitless and we end up having to order one which won't be in until tomorrow.

I'm already starting to get agitated when the accountant gets in touch to tell us there's a cheque book stub missing. So, it's off to the piles and files in search of it, poor Simon once again mucking in to search for something that I appear to have misplaced and am caught up in a growing spiral of panic about, whilst none of our 'real' work is getting done. Finally, the accountant calls again, delighted to say that I sent it with the rest of the paperwork that he'd needed to do the VAT return. I don't know what to make of this information. I have no recollection whatsoever of putting the stub in, goodness, if I'd even had an inkling I'd have been on the phone to get *him* checking through paperwork, instead of letting us perform the wild goose chase here.

I'm exhausted and stressed. I can feel it coursing through my veins and start to settle, in the furrows of my brow. It's just on 2pm and I know I've hit my wall: I can't take any more so I ask Antony to run us home. He's affable about it and, in truth, probably glad to be left to get on in peace, so we're home before half past, for a light lunch and a bit of alone-time before Simon has to go and get his train.

It's lovely spending this little hiatus and although I'm happy that Simon has his own life, his wife and is happy and settled, I'm sad to see him go. I won't be on my own tonight though because Antony's staying over as he's going to work again tomorrow. He arrives after shutting up the business for the night, signalling time to take Simon to the station, so I come too, to say goodbye.

When it comes to it though, I can't do the whole seeing him off on the train thing. I hate all this going away. Since January I now have this awful disquiet, this sense that now I can never feel sure of when I will see people again, which gives rise to all the old fear from hospital, all those days when the rancid terrors were just running through my body, leaving me helpless in their wake: they'll have their way, one day and they rise occasionally, like today, to remind me so, leaving me unnerved, terrified and very lonely. So, to wait for the train with Simon is too much and instead we leave him at the station.

The issue of supper arises and, partly for a change and partly, I think, because he knows I'm not myself, Antony suggests we stop by the fish and chip shop on the way home. A supper like this is real comfort food and a rare treat for me, a deviation from my juice and clean diet. In all honesty, with the different visitors and company of the least few weeks, I have slipped a bit but now, with the steroids reducing and with the fact that I have lost a stone in weight since, I feel that maybe it is good for me to be less careful for a change, especially on a day like today. So, although I know I am happier when I stay on the clean diet, I also know that tonight is an exception, so fish and chips it is!

#

I'm feeling a little better today. Simon texts to say that he's arrived home safely, thank God, although he had a rough old flight.

It's Sam and Simon's anniversary today, so I send them an early text to wish them a happy day before setting off to work with Antony. I think I'm doing a little better on the admin side today, I'm still not as productive as I used to be, my routines still slow and laborious, but I'm getting there today.

I take an hour out to go to an acupuncture session, then wander back to work, stopping off at the bakery to pick up some lunch. This feels like the old me a little, getting on, doing things, taking it all in my stride.

When I arrive back at work I settle to my lunch and decide to check my phone, to see if Sam got my text. I get the first cold grasp of anxiety as I realise that I no longer have my mobile and what's more, I have no idea where it is. Antony obviously sees the agitation building in me and very kindly retraces my steps for me, back to the bakery and then to the Holistic Centre, but no one at either place has seen it.

By now, I'm really starting to feel upset. This isn't the kind of thing where you shrug and say, oh well, get another one. My phone's more to me than that: it's my last means of contact with people other than e-mail and I have lots of things stored on there which I just don't know if I could track down or remember without it.

I'm supposed to be going to the supermarket after work for a few bits and to buy a voucher I want to get for Sam, but I'm finding it hard to concentrate, to think beyond what I'll do, what I'll be without my phone. The new stapler arrives, which should be a practical distraction, but I can't get it to work, the staple holder just keeps shooting out whenever I press it, so I don't know what to do about that either. Antony has a go and I'm not sure if I'm pleased or annoyed that it does the same for him. OK, so it's not me being useless with it, but it does mean we've waited for a broken stapler to arrive and now we still can't get the dispatches done.

I'm also feeling extra anxious, but of course can't explain to Antony why, but this week has been a terror for the double-incontinence. This most disturbing and unpredictable condition adds an extra dimension to stressful days, having the effect of just when you think things can't get any worse, there's suddenly crap in all senses of the word to deal with. It's not helping the day and the day isn't helping the condition.

It's a joint decision to give the day up as a bad job. Antony takes me to the supermarket and wanders around amiably whilst I follow my list around the shop. As we arrive at the checkout, his mobile starts to ring – it's the holistic centre to say they've found my phone under a chair! Well, I'm almost faint with relief but before I can start to share this with Antony, the man behind us in the queue taps me on the shoulder and says, "did you lose your ring?"

In his hand he's holding my little marcasite ring. Of course I tell him that it's mine, but that I thought I lost it on a visit to the old town on Monday. Antony's sure that it's just fallen out of my pocket, but I know I checked it thoroughly, I just know I did! We finish up in the supermarket and I can't stop beaming as Antony stops by the holistic centre to pick up my phone, before dropping me back home.

So, it's been a strange kind of a day. They say these things are sent to try, and I do feel exceedingly tried and tested, and of course exhausted as a result. But exhaustion has its compensations: I'm far too tired to ponder the hows of the loss and reappearance of both my ring and my mobile, instead I just accept the warm and happy comfort of knowing that they have both come back to me. I also accept that I'm happy to be at home and can think of nothing nicer, at this particular moment, than my bed. It's only 7.30 but the day feels like a long one, so I'm heading off for an early night.

#

It's something of a shock to realise that we're almost at the end of this 'holiday' month. Even though I've been nowhere, I've had plenty of visitors and today it's the turn of my old friend Catherine, from London. She's my school gate friend, as I call her, and I look forward to seeing her with that sense of anticipation and reconnection which comes automatically when you've known someone as long as we have, which is about 30 years in all. We've always managed to strike that balance of being there for each other without living in each other's pockets.

When I open the door to her we hug as if holding each other up and she says that she had no idea what to expect when seeing me today. The last time she saw me was during my first ten days in hospital. Apparently I'd not only mostly failed to recognise her, I'd also commented to Sam that her talking was getting on my nerves, even referring to her, one of my very best friends, as "that woman"! How thankful I am that she's forgiving and totally understanding of the fact that I really wasn't myself and even if I'm not fully back to how I was, at least I'm not *that* person any more!

We spend a lovely day catching up. She says she's surprised at how much I have improved, clearly impressed that I can now manage in the house without a stick. We are able to go to town for lunch and have a slow walk on the beach, another plus for both of us and such a relief for her I think. I do get the impression that she may have been expecting to be visiting someone more of an invalid than the person who is now in front of her. It makes me glad to have exceeded someone's expectations, even if I don't really meet my own, quite a bit of the time.

Of course there are limits to how fabulous I can be at one sitting! By this evening, I'm overcome with exhaustion: the tinnitus has seemed so loud today and I feel I've had to work so hard to hear and to be clear myself when speaking. I can't begin to explain the effort involved in being with someone all day and although it's worth it to me, to catch up with a lovely friend who I've not seen for so long, it's truly wiped me out. As the clock inches towards 9pm I know I can't stay up a moment longer, so I say goodnight and leave her watching the telly before her own bedtime.

So now I lay me down to sleep and it stresses me entirely that for all Catherine sees improvement upon improvement, I just get so tired so very easily just by doing what I used to enjoy, with my anxiety levels rising all the time as I'm faced with the menaces of my condition and the huge question each time of whether I'll be able to cope, whether I'll be able to enjoy this time.

#

Catherine leaves at 9.30 next morning, after what has been a very lovely visit. Yes, I have coped and yes, I'm still very tired. I've taken this morning off, not in the work sense, more in the 'being' sense. I ignore my list of chores, all the glaring jobs I spy around the house and take it easy, just doing a bit of tidying as and when I feel like it. I'm trying to conserve my energies a bit, not just from yesterday but because I'm also having lunch with an old friend later. That's probably poor planning on my part, to have two main events on consecutive days but, as I'm sure I've said, I'm finding it imperative to catch up with people who are important to me, especially those I don't see so often because I just don't know what the future holds and, not to be morbid but in the context of the thief just pragmatic, who knows when *this* time is the last time?

Thankfully I don't have to go out. John's coming here to eat. He's a good friend, we studied for our degree together from 2000 to 2004 and have continued to keep in touch ever since. We'd always meet up every couple of months for lunch and a bottle of wine but of course since I've been indisposed those months since our last lunch have stretch out across almost a year. Goodness, so much has changed!

As he crosses the threshold I burst into tears as he's truly one of the people I wondered if I would ever see again. I continue to cry but also laugh as we settle to lunch and catching up, just like old times. He talks about his voluntary work and his private practice but mainly wants to know about my illness, he seems genuinely interested and horrified in equal measures! He then tells me of a friend's friend who also had the virus some time ago and that it took him 18 months to get back to full time work – a whole 18 months! I guess that gives me a more realistic idea of how long I might be looking at for my full recovery, although I know of course that no two people are the same, nor are they necessarily left in the same state following the Encephalitis itself.

It's easy talking to John, but it's also easy listening to him too. John's father was also deaf and afflicted with tinnitus so, like Frances in her professional role, John can not only empathise with me, he also uses strategies to help me not to miss any snippets of our conversation, which makes a real difference to me. I feel like I'm in a proper dialogue, not a part dialogue, part monologue where I'm saying to myself, "what was that? What's he saying? I wish he'd move his hand from his mouth so I can see his lips more clearly" … and all that.

After a nice lunch and a lovely time he has to leave to get his train back to Brighton. It seems so soon and the house now seems very quiet and tranquil. I settle down to do some writing, to be still and calm like the rest of the house.

A little while later I stand up to get a pen and to my surprise I catch two little faces outside the window, arms waving at me ... Sam and Evie on their way home from France! Oh joy of joys to see them, it's the perfect round off to my month of visitors. In they come, Simon too and we all have supper together. They all look so well and Evie, well she seems so big and less of a baby and more of a little girl now, it's amazing the difference that a couple of weeks out of sight (but not out of mind, of course) can make! They stay until it's time to get going and get Evie settled. Of course, what they don't know is that it's just about my bedtime too, so once they are on their way, I batten down the hatches and then climb up the stairs to bed, glad to know that my children are all safe and sound.

#

As usually happens, I'm paying for all my activities with exhaustion and body pain today. It doesn't help that when I was up for my usual round of toileting in the night, I then couldn't get back to sleep. So, at 3am I was up looking for a book to settle back down with. I then saw the clock again at 4 something and then again at 6ish.

I'm invited to Sam and Simon's for a breakfast of croissants they brought from France so Simon arrives at about 10am to pick me up. It's lovely to spend time with them after so long and to play with Evie whilst they catch up on their gardening and of course the mountains of holiday laundry. I feel useful and wanted and I'm genuinely happy to be here with them.

Unfortunately though, the incontinence is extremely bad today. It's such an intrusion in my life, along with everything else, yet has the unique factor of being the one thing that no-one, even me, really wants to talk about. I can't think about it without crying, much less talk about it without the emotions and despair creeping in. By lunchtime it's intolerable and I feel horribly uncomfortable and I'm getting really agitated about odours, so I ask to come home again. I am better at home where I can cope with frequent changing and just manage myself better really.

I collapse, exhausted onto the sofa after yet another change, and I catch fleeting movement once again out of the corners of my eyes. I don't know if there is any connection but the rats in my head are back again, in the chimney, in the fireplace. I know they are there, but of course they never fully appear, not properly, just half formed, like me.

#

I've just realised that all this time that I have been caught up in my world there have been Olympics that I can't hear. Now and then I catch highlights on the telly and see little snippets, but it holds none of the interest for me that I would have expected. I have no enthusiasm for it, I just don't feel it.

#

It's the final Sunday of August. Today I wakened to a lovely bright morning at 6.30, so I did the usual of coming down for porridge, then back to bed to read for a while. To tell the truth, I don't want to get up today, I just want to stay put, so I do so until after 8am, when I have to push myself to get going so that I won't be late for Mass.

As I get up and go through my routine of washing and dressing, I'm overcome with a sadness that makes my arms too heavy to slip into sleeves, my body too hunched to unfurl into clothing. Tears aren't far away, I feel them tickling my eyes, my cheeks. I ask myself what I want, what's wrong with me? I hear myself answer that I just want my children home, here with me. I almost think of them as little ones that I want to look after and protect instead of as the capable independent adults that they are, with their own families and responsibilities. I don't really remember, or acknowledge that they don't really need me now, they have formed their own families and support systems. I've fulfilled my motherly role and it's as it should be, but I miss them and somehow, for some reason today, I'm grieving for those times.

#

Sam and Simon pick me up from Mass and I make myself useful by doing some ironing for them and playing with Evie, which is of course never a chore but a joy! I'm having a lovely time and it's a wrench to come away, but I do so in plenty of time: keeping it short is still the secret to getting on well I think and so it's what I do. I can see that our relationship has improved since they had a holiday so the break has definitely done them good – both the holiday and the break from me, I guess. I don't want to be a burden to them, or to anyone and I still maintain as I have said before that I'd rather they didn't do things for me rather than resent what they do, or feel they have to appear willing. I know better than anyone how hard it is to keep with that kind of appearance.

18. Encephalitis Recovery: A Pregnant Pause

September starts with a very busy day: my first appointment since what seems like forever with the neurologist. In between appointments I keep my list, jotting down questions as I think of things to ask him once the appointment comes round again. I updated it last night and found that I now have 37 questions!

Of course, in the period of time since the last appointment, some of those earlier questions aren't really relevant, but I keep them there and highlight the new questions, so I can be sure of asking. Being sure is so important to me now.

It's kind of a medical day really, as I have to pop into the doctor's surgery first to pick up my repeat prescription, but of course when I get there there's an item which isn't due yet, so I'll have to come back again next week for that one.

A quick stop off at the pharmacy to pick up my meds then I have to go into the office on the way to the hospital. This popping into work is a bit of a strange one as I know I'm not going to be working; on the contrary, I'm checking for the arrival of some important post I've been expecting, the return of a confidentiality letter sent out to one of the people who have expressed an interest in the sale of the company. If this letter's back, I can send out the packs I've prepared: three year's accounts, company brochure, local Business Link Review and company resume. It's taken me weeks to prepare this information so finding the confidentiality letter has come today brings mixed feelings: of fear versus excitement; practical versus emotional. In any case, it means that my work in these preparations hasn't been in vain but, as I send the materials off, I realise that I'm now at the start of a longer process or is that a shorter one, which takes me to the next phase of my life - and who knows what state I'll be in by then?

Hopefully the hospital will have some of the answers and it's here that the next few hours of my day are spent. The usual routine ensues: sit and wait in chairs for a bit, before the nurse takes me into her room and weighs me. She is talking, animatedly, probably cheerily but as she's mostly turned away from me, scrawling her findings onto my notes for the neurologist, I just can't hear her. I go through the explanation of being deaf and explain that I need to see her face when she speaks.

She weighs me and converts the kilos into pounds, before calculating on her fingers then telling me I have lost 12 lb since June. She does face me as she tells me this and wonders why I've lost this weight. I explain to her that I think it is because it takes so much energy to do things, living at home. I also explain that I now have different eating habits, with smaller, easily managed meals and that I stick to a clean diet with plenty of juicing, in fact I don't eat much sweet stuff, like cakes and biscuits at all now.

Then it's another short wait in the corridor until the neurologist calls me in. He says very little but I feel he is assessing me from the minute he comes to his door. He watches me walk into his room and how I sit down. He too asks about my weight and I give the same explanation before we launch into the real stuff. We both know I'm not here about my weight, for goodness sake.

Everything else we talk about has been touched on before and the standard answer is usually that it's "due to the medicine." However, now that the steroids have been reducing (and that's been going well) he says that we can reduce them farther still, by another 5mg, bringing me down to 10mg daily. It's fascinating that this seems to have changed everything. This time, as we go through my list everything, from my hot-freezing legs to the fact of wearing incontinence pads for the better part of a year causing me pain to sit, is all now referred to as "part of the condition."

Despite this new and to be honest not very hopeful information that the incontinence now falls under the banner of being "part of the condition" I pursue the issue. It may be part and parcel of a condition to him, but for me it's part, parcel and damned pad of my day to day existence and I've just about had enough. I try to explain how uncomfortable it is wearing pads all the time; it was always pretty bad but now, having lost a stone in weight overall, when I sit down it is truly painful, I feel like my iscial tuberosity (those sitting bones) are going to come through my skin. He's sympathetic but can only assure me that, yes, it's all part of the condition.

When I tell him I am still emotional, he tells me to stick with the clinical psychologist, but he doesn't seem to appreciate that the lack of availability is difficult – sometimes it can be a whole month between appointments. Yes, I expect that's better than nothing but in reality it's not good enough. I feel it welling up in me and I'm really not sure whether I'm going to burst into tears or temper. I tell him I was so upset about the length of time it took before I was able to move back to my own home, having been told if I went to my daughter's for a fortnight's recovery then I could go home. I try to explain that somehow I thought those two weeks would be my recovery time. Anyway, here we are nine months later overall and I've been home for about six or seven weeks. He acknowledges that "with this condition" recovery times can be too difficult to predict - another way of gently telling me that the slow recovery is all part of the condition too. In fact, the answers to most of my questions are agreements really or that it's to do with the condition.

I share that I'm trying to sell the business and he agrees that it seems like a good idea, all things considered.

I do tell him that my confidence is growing, that I can feel it myself and, sometimes within those moments, catch a glimpse of my old self and I know that our appointment is coming to a close. He concludes with a comment about my referral to London for my hearing and also confirms that another MRI scan will be done in the New Year. Our time is clearly over, so I don't bother to ask my last question, about flying. Although I'd love to fly over to visit my family in Ireland, making such a journey is not my priority right now. Although I think this has been a good appointment in all, one thing I've picked up today is that I'm still very much in the recovery phase. It feels ironic, after nine long months, just like a pregnancy, to still be in "my condition."

#

So, day to day it stays the same in my head, a constant routine of just trying to remember what has to be done. The week still starts with a list of what is on every day - there is nothing else in there apart from what's to be done, there's no extras, no real knowledge or information, delightful snippets of my own to bring to the party.

My sister tells me she has been to see some singer and tells me her name. I know I'm supposed to respond favourably to this, but I have no idea who she's on about. So, I ask all about it, hopeful of gleaning the information I need.

"Where's she from?"

"England, she's English."

"What does she sing?"

"Ah, you know, you know her!"

"No, I don't." The old me may have done, but this is me, now.

"Yes, you do. She was big in the theatre ... Miss Saigon, Blood Brothers ..."

"What was her name again?"

"Barbara Dickson."

"No, I have no recollection of that name."

"Of course you know her, of course you do!"

So, of course I do, of course I know, of course I remember. Despite all this time, it's just like those early days in the hospital - all of that information's just wiped away and no one offers an understanding of my not knowing, no comprehension of how everything I might have known and understood, has just been wiped out.

#

The slight difference now is that, to some extent, I can now read for information. I've slowly regained my ability to read, but it's mechanical and automatic, a perfunctory process which tires me out and leaves me empty, as I have no memory of what the content is. On a good day I can read, digest and reflect for just a moment, then the content is once more lost to me.

After all this time and even in the context of the other awful struggles, such as the heat of the summer and the darned incontinence; I find that I'm currently struggling so much more with the memory loss. The difficulty with the memory loss is that it's not apparent – I can be engaged with the person I am talking to, listening attentively and then – well then there's nothing else. I'm in the moment, just this moment right now, but then there's nothing else. Except for my lists. My lists are my thinking aloud and seem to go on and on, thoughts committed before being lost, instructions given before being forgotten. I sometimes despair of ever feeling right again.

#

The photos in the hallway still haunt me, by the way. Faces I can't place. Instead I consider other photos, baby photos that I'm certain have hung on my wall for years but are now nowhere to be found. I check my walls in case I'm remembering the walls themselves wrongly, maybe I'm in the wrong place or perhaps they are? But the baby photos are gone. I am heartbroken but they are lost.

#

I finally decide to follow up with the name of the other Encephalitis survivor that my physio has treated in the past - now that I have her number again, I guess it's time I actually called her.

I feel a little nervous and self-conscious, but this does seem like one of the very few opportunities I've had to actually talk things through with someone who really does understand what it's like. So, I put on my aids, turn the loudspeaker up on the phone and … here goes.

She answers after a short time and sounds very nice, very upbeat and not at all phased by my call. She explains that she had the illness in 1984 and has been left with severe residual lack of abilities, for example, when walking, she actually has to use a wheelchair quite a lot. At the time, she says, she was so ill she was in a coma and was paralysed after diagnosis, so she was transferred to a neurological hospital.

She tells me, "of course we could be dead! Did you know that one in five die?"

I can't help the thought that rushes in here, of how many times I've thought about the fact that if I'd died I wouldn't have had to go through all this recovery, this incontinence, this lack of physical and emotional control. As if she can read my mind, she adds that she has little control over her emotions … she can either burst out laughing or crying at the drop of a hat.

At length, when she has told her story, she asks if the same things happened to me. I tell her straight, no, I wasn't in a coma or paralysed but I explain that I've been so very debilitated, even when I was discharged from hospital and am still struggling in so many areas.

"Well," she says, "it wasn't very serious then."

As graciously as I can muster, I point out that it's now nine months since January when I was taken to hospital, that I'm still struggling to regain a lot of my abilities and strength so, on the contrary, it all seems pretty serious to me.

I divert the conversation slightly, by talking about how hard my illness has been for my children.

"Mine were OK," she shared, "but of course they've been brought up well and learned to stand on their own two feet, not hang onto my apron strings."

I feel inordinately upset and incredibly dismissed, yet this woman is the only link I have with someone who has really experienced this, so we agree that we might meet up next month. As I replace the phone, I don't feel stronger for having forged a link with this woman, I feel weaker, like I've been judged and, once again, been found lacking. I know that I won't meet up with her.

#

Of course, the joy of another hydrotherapy session arrives but the physio is concerned. She says I'm not as strong as I should be and she gives me a tough workout in the pool, which is exhausting beyond belief. I almost don't have the strength left to dry and dress myself, but sit, wrapped and dripping in my towel in the changing cubicle until I can muster my tired limbs into the action required.

She's also concerned about my weight loss and asks me if I want to see a nutritionist. I tell her that the nutritionist contacted me on discharge but because of my hearing I missed her call, so I wrote and asked her to contact me again and wouldn't you know, I'm still waiting!

As I leave, the physio notices that I've painted my nails, for just the second time since I was discharged. She declares this a good sign of my on-going progress: yet another kind and well-meaning professional who looks to the outer, deceiving signs for reassurance, whilst I feel myself crumbling and failing inside.

#

I'm doing quite a bit where I can and realise that on the face of it, some of my achievements show remarkable progress indeed. In this month alone I've had days where:

- I've gone from the GP, to work, to hospital.
- I've been at work then gone off to hydro.
- I've been at work then taken a cab to the supermarket, done my shopping and then taken a cab home. That's the first time I've done it both ways

with no help, no permission and my time was my own, independently.

However, it's easy to look at that list and think, well there she goes, on her feet, independent, back to normal. But the truth is I still wear the Emperor's new clothes for the majority of my outings. Like that work and shopping day, it really wasn't easy for me but I did it nonetheless. I was so anxious about it and although I was out there, independently at it, Christina was in the office so she called me a cab, which was a help and of course it helps me enormously to feel that I have that kind of back up.

This is the thing about ABI or the condition for me, the fact that it just doesn't show. I look 'normal' so to speak and the bits that I know are not my normal are all concealed: the freezing legs; the burning feet; the incontinence; the body pain; the loss of abilities; the loss of hearing; the loss of memory, no driving, no flying; no ability to watch TV or listen to the radio, much less go to a concert; being unable to use the phone easily; now unable to sing ... I could go on, but really, I'm sick of this list so I'm sure everyone else must be.

So, to those who pass me in the shops, those who see me out and about, those who read my journal entries of a week full of medical visits and chores, it sounds like I'm just carrying out a normal week, at least within some contexts. But if you consider that up to January 2008 I was working full time, spent lots of time with my family and still fitted in social events and hobbies it makes me again aware of my loss of energy and the excruciating length of time it takes me to do even the simplest things.

#

Its strange how things change and how priorities alter. My priority pre-Encephalitis was to be a good grandma, helpful and supportive, although I'd had to say that I couldn't offer any child care as I would still need to work to support myself. But that was fine, I was told that I wasn't expected to as Sam would go back to work part-time and that they'd decided to use a nursery a couple of days a week, so that was all set.

Yes, it had been part of my thinking to sell off my business eventually but not yet, certainly not yet. It was a dream for the future, when I'd be financially secure and then free to spend time with my son and his wife, visit with my sisters for more than just a few days at a time, concentrate on my project work at the counselling centre and go off on my travels. However, I'd fully anticipated that for the first six months to a year of my official retirement from the business, I'd do what I really wanted to do, which is to help Sam with Evie and visit my son Simon.

Of course, my wishes to do these things are sill there but the priority now is to be *well enough* to do them. I feel tired just trying to get myself well, which is like a full-time job in itself, there is so much to do: get exercise; take a walk, take medicine; boil herbs; eat three meals a day; add in hospital appointments for neurology, psychology, hydro and occasionally (or should that be intermittently?) hearing and that is enough in itself, without housework and the garden.

Then there's the not being able to do some of the jobs, which presents a whole other challenge. Just thinking of ways around this is often more tiring than if I'd been able to just get on and do them myself; thinking about them and not being able to do them is very tiring.

So, nine months on from the Encephalitis, my pregnant pause, I'm still awaiting my recovery, my rebirth.

#

Happily, things have continued to improve between Sam and myself. I am still convinced the secret is the short visits and I don't ask her to do much. At the moment I'm mindful of the fact that she's only been back to work for a week or so, since the long summer holidays, which I know is a wrench for her after having some lovely, quality time at home with Evie. Tonight they've come for dinner and everyone's happy and relaxed because it's a Friday night and the weekend stretches ahead, luxurious and long. It's lovely to see them so relaxed here, it reminds me of when they came around when Simon visited and they were all together. I guess this means that this is just the second time I've cooked properly for them since January. And this, after what feels like a long week of doing things myself, for myself, by myself, so I allow myself the slightly delighted feeling that I too have earned my Friday night! They don't want to keep Evie out too late but to be honest we're all so relaxed and companionable that it's around 9 before they leave, which is lovely. After they've said goodnight, I make the most of this relaxed feeling by popping my sleeping tablet and taking myself off to bed too.

#

Saturdays of course are chore days, so I've spent the morning doing chores. In the process, I've made quite a bit of mess, looking through and sorting things, so the place is pretty untidy but it's all work in progress as far as I'm concerned.

Sam pops in with Evie, to say hello and thanks for last night, but she's hardly sat down in the lounge – the scene of my current splurge in progress - before she offers to hoover, telling me the room needs it.

"No thanks," I say. "It'll get done when I'm finished."

Instead, I ask her to carry the ironing upstairs for me, which she does. In the process she notices that I have things on the stairs, so she starts to put them away. I know she's trying to be helpful but I feel agitated and have to ask her not to and try to explain that they're part of the work in progress, to remind me about specific jobs and if they're not there then I'll forget that I have these jobs to do. I can tell she's affronted, whether it's by the state of my house, the fact I don't want the help for the moment or just the fact that I can't be swayed from my routine which keeps me organised (however disorganised it appears to others). I just don't know, but there's definitely a tension now which, even once they leave, stays with me.

In fact, it's still very much part of today, Sunday. I'm trying to read the newspaper but my mind keeps wandering to Sam's comment about the room needing hovering and a few other bits I had mentioned that were poo-pooed. Before I realise it, I again have tears running down my face as I'm wracked with wretchedness and a feeling that once more I've been criticised, judged and found to be wanting.

Sam texts to say she is not going to Mass but is going to Tunbridge Wells instead. She asks if I'm ok and whether I want a lift to Mass anyway. I text back that I'm OK and no thanks to the lift, I'm still getting ready for Mass. So I haul myself out of my wallow and start to get ready. I'm just about there when the doorbell rings.

Sam stands there, saying she got a sense from my text that all was not well with me so she's here to check. Inside the house, I tell her that I felt criticised. I tell her that I just want to say this, get it off my chest but don't want to get into a discussion. She agrees and says that it was not meant as criticism, it was just an offering to help. I share with her that her intention might have been helpful, but her tone was not.

After she leaves, I'm in pieces again. No matter how I try to manage myself, my own self-management seems to be in question. I said I didn't want a lift but she still came round although in truth I was trying to avoid meeting her until my feelings are more settled, until I've got over this little blip in my head, but she can't seem to leave things. I guess I need to be clearer with her, to assert myself and be able to say I don't want a lift thanks and do not come round just now. I truly hope that, as my confidence grows, I will be better able to deal with this stuff and that it need not be such a threat to our relationship. So for now I just continue to cry, the luxury of the weekend now scattered in sodden tissues around me.

#

Today I get a letter from DVLA to say I can drive again. It is another link in the chain of events, of things coming together. Hmm, although now I suppose I will have to notify them of my being deaf. I think I'll leave that for another day ... it's not like I'm intending jumping back into the driving seat anytime soon!

#

I have another sisterly visit, this time two together, Grainne and Sheila. I'm delighted they're here, but I must say that I'm finding having two visitors a bit too much from the point of communication, whereas one at a time I can cope with. Grainne is extremely good and is naturally astute at making sure I can access what's going on - she touches my arm to get my attention before speaking and then she speaks slowly. She also seems calmer, clearer somehow.

I'm finding it trickier to communicate with Sheila. It's hard to get her to understand that if I can't see her face, then it's so much harder for me to hear her. She continues to speak to me when she's behind me or she's busy doing something else at the same time. I find myself repeating to her, "I need to see your face" after which she'll then really raise her voice, come very close to my face and with exaggerated facial movements say "what I was saying was

..." I'm finding this very difficult, although I can see its comedy value. I can also see how hard it is for them to adapt too, after all, we've had our ways of carrying on and gabbing on with each other since childhood, they are used to a me who was able to hear, not this me, who can't.

They don't really comment on my illness and although there are aspects of this I'm grateful for, I would also welcome the chance for a sympathetic ear to talk it through with. So they don't really ask how I'm doing either, but I guess this is mainly because, once I started to be less of a chimp back at the computer, we've kept up-to-date mainly by e-mail.

Of course, whilst they're here they want to be useful but I've found a lot of the weekend difficult. I know they're trying to help when they take my stick or my bag and hold onto it whilst I'm trying to juggle it to where I want it. The trouble is, not asking if I want help is just that automatic mother to child reaction and something which brings out the worst in even the old me, let alone the more forthright new me. I want to revolt against it and shout out "I'm deaf, not stupid but even with the deafness you could still ask what I want, if I want something and, very specifically, if I want *help* with something."

Grainne says she's astounded at my hearing loss and how difficult it is for me to hear, but apart from this they don't show any feeling or opinion about the state of me, so I don't know what they are thinking now. Sheila says she knows a woman who had Encephalitis some years ago who made a full recovery, but she has not read about the ones who have not. I'm kind of reminded about that other woman on the end of the phone, with her one in five statistics. I'm not sure what it means that there are statistics for dying from it but few for recovery. Please God I am going to make a full recovery, although no one can tell me for sure that I will, they say "should", the best they can offer me.

#

Sam's been on a course today and she calls by on her way home. She has a heavy cold, you can see it in her eyes that she's tired and feeling very low. She seems to be upset about a lot of things and isn't sure why. Bless her, I think she has time to think about herself a little at the moment and this isn't in fact a positive for her: she never does well when she is not under pressure and she bothers me for sure when she's like this. I don't know what to say that's right, because she latches on to one thing I say and then makes a meal of it, even if it was just meant as a conversational, throw-away remark.

So, we talk about her aunties' visit and my progress yet she almost seems upset that I am not as dependent on her as I have been, whilst at the same time she tells me that she is pleased and proud of how well I have got on and progressed in my recovery. We'd hug but she doesn't want to pass on her cold, so we kind of pat each other, which says nothing and everything, really.

#

So to the end of another month. And the upshot of it, of all my progress? I'm embarrassed, almost ashamed that it's coming up to the end of the ninth month of the year and I've still had not made a full recovery. Of course, this impatience, like the thief, rats and ghouls is mine alone as others constantly tell me how well they think I am doing.

#

I feel sad for my children that I am not what I thought I would be by now, for me or for them. I have to remind myself that I did not choose this disease or this situation but I feel that I ought to be able to speed up my recovery somehow. In reality though, I'm doing absolutely everything that is suggested recommended or prescribed and then some. So I have to accept that perhaps time is the healer and I can't hurry time. Unbelievably we're nine months in and I'm just discovering the truth: to get better I have to be *patient* patient.

19. Attitudes and Platitudes or, What Not to Say to Someone Recovering from Encephalitis

Yes, there are plenty of days which are tougher than others, but more often than not I'm finding that it's not "just" the physicality or even the psychological aspects of what's happened (and in truth is still happening) which gets me down the most. Despite all of that, these awful, relentless symptoms, reminders of the thief's visit, what gets me down the most is that no-one else seems to realise the extent of what this illness is, or truly recognise what it's actually done to me. My children, friends, my siblings, indeed any and all of those who visit me regularly have little or no knowledge of Encephalitis – nor of any other Acquired Brain Injury for that matter.

Although of course they're not to blame for this in themselves, the fact is there's a real gap out there. Or is it in here, in this world I find myself in? Whichever way you look at it, I've come to realise there's just a real absence of training in how to deal with the Encephalitis recovery, this emotional and physical aftermath as well as its ABI legacy. What's more, this gap isn't just evident as part of my journey and my need for support, it's also evident in what others need in order to be able to support me. Without it, our attempts are based at best on good intentions which, in the event, just aren't good enough.

#

"Aren't you doing well?" This, because I'm appearing in public and thus appearing to manage is the number one comment I hate. There's no recognition of the difference in the shape of my being, the lapsed routine of my days, the shallow pool of day-to-day energy, from which these appearances are drawn, the remainder of which goes into making a meal, pushing the vacuum about (which I have to admit I fail miserably at) or wearily loading the washing machine. I still cry without any thought for why I am crying and I'm still expected to account for this, the unaccountable condition I find myself in and a personal reaction to it that I can't justify, but shouldn't really be expected to explain.

#

Even as time moves on, as I'm making progress, there's still a significant reluctance of others to believe what I tell them of my condition, of my progress.

For example, I can express a wish to get better, that is to say, better than I am at this moment. In response to this, I'm cheerily told about someone's friend who made a complete recovery or am dismissed with "you're doing fine".

And am I fine with that? As I learned a long time back in Transactional Analysis, others feel they're rescuing you with their helpful words, largely because they just can't listen to what's being said and sit with it, they need to fill the space or try to reassure you with their own theory on how it is. This, sadly, is of no help to me. Instead it just adds to the list of things to cope with: there's a certain pressure which comes with knowing that so-and-so made a complete recovery at a certain stage, an inference that perhaps I should have too, by now?

This reassurance also smacks far more of what others want to believe for their own comfort. It removes their need to have to hear how things really are for me, better for them to tell themselves I'm "doing fine."

And how about that: "you're doing fine"? This words fall upon my Encephalitic deaf ears with an alternative meaning. I hear them as: "we all just have to get on with it." It may be true, of course and yes, some are better able to rise to that challenge than others (and let's be in no doubt here, it is a serious challenge), I think, whilst others may have less to cope with in the "getting on with it."

In short, I experience such platitudes as a lack of acceptance:

* From those who haven't had the illness, because they can't comprehend the impact of it, or cope with facing up to the "could happen to any of us" reality that Viral Encephalitis presents. These are the individuals who see me up and about as a reflection of my being "fine." They ignore the visible signs of disability, like the sticks and the hearing aids: so long as I'm up and at it, I'm recovered.

* From those who have been acquainted with the illness, usually once or twice removed, the whole friend-of-a-friend brigade. Their "experience" of

someone else's reality gives them a standpoint from which to compare and to judge me.

* From those who have had the illness. Like that awful other patient, who judged me as not being seriously ill because, thanks possibly to my timely visit to Dr. Shen as the virus was trying to get a hold and definitely thanks to the pro-activity of my daughter in getting medical assistance, I didn't end up in a coma. That means I've had it easy, apparently.

#

It's not until I finally start to spend time with individuals from the Encephalitis Society that I start to realise that such platitudes and lack of acceptance all across the board is part of what's holding me back from being able to accept my condition myself. An attitude problem all of my own.

#

I think of my confidence as mobile, an entity somewhat quicker on its feet than I am. It's certainly a false confidence. When I have company or am in familiar settings and surroundings, my confidence goes up and I feel good, supported and capable. But when these scaffolds fall away or are absent, my confidence drops and I am lost once again, in some kind of abyss of fear which seems deep and endless. I know this can happen to anybody from time to time but I know that for me, before Encephalitis, its depth was barely down ever, let alone on most occasions, like now. Of course my confidence was occasionally misplaced, anyone who's ever been divorced will understand that … but completely sapped? Never. Yet now, when I'm in an unfamiliar place and can't find the stairs to the loo, or which door to go out or in, the feeling that consumes me. And these are just the basics, of course, the day-to-day that I have no confidence in. So when people say, "but you're doing so well!" they have no idea just how badly I'm doing, on the inside.

For sure part of this is because many of my props and prompts are so hidden. Any and all of my days out are fully prompted by visual aids and my infernal bloody list-making. One of these days when a friend and I go out, is a good example. I go out and check my list, I have visual reminders: a cash machine and a hardware shop, to remind me to withdraw cash and there is a sink plug on the list. My props serve me well, so I'm told "Well ... there's nothing wrong with your memory!"

Maybe I should feel like a child, patted on the head but I don't, I feel so angry I could cuss. I want to scream: "No? So when I crossed the courtyard for the Ladies, why was I so scared that I wouldn't be able to find the restaurant I had just left you sitting in?"

#

I'm more reflective at the moment and I know that I have real frustrations with the lack of understanding that seems to come from those around me, even though I do know that none of this is calculated or deliberate.

My sister seems to think that a lot of these things that have come up are unresolved issues from the past. However, at last, I seem to have regained the ability to create an opinion all of my very own and, in the truth of my own opinion, I don't necessarily agree with her. She says that living in England has me exiled from my childhood, my family, which raises feelings of isolation and loss, but I know I don't really think or feel that.

Living in England was a choice I made and I now know that I have no wish to live in Ireland, although I did think about it briefly when I was in my twenties. At that time we also talked about going to Australia but I settled well here in England and I've built my life here since so no, I don't feel exiled or isolated. I don't know why I have hung on to these particular memories, when others slipped away with the thief but here they are. Perhaps this bit of knowledge helps me to protect my family, my Irish past, so don't say this situation's a result of any of that, just don't. I won't have it blamed for how I feel now, the crying, the loneliness, the isolation; this doesn't reflect Ireland's absence, it reflects the thief's presence.

#

In amongst my copious lists, I'm compiling one detailing the worst things to say to someone who's had / is still struggling with Encephalitis. Of course it's a personal list, based on my experiences and as far as platitudes go, these are the ones guaranteed to bring out my very worst frustrations:

"*Think positive*" or "*just put it behind you, let it go*" – from GP, to consultants, to family and friends. If being positive made you better I'd have made a full recovery, wouldn't I? Constantly being told to think positive, to just let it go seems to be a stock response when I say I am going to try something new.

The thing is, it's because I'm on the inside of this body and they're on the outside. Of course I am the one looking for answers and solutions which maybe not in accordance with their wishes, their belief systems or their standards in this, my play for life, my quest for damage limitation, my overwhelming need to regain some of what was lost. I truly wonder, not in the bitchy sense, but in the full amazed wonderment sense, how they would react should it be them, looking for the way to put their lives back together again? *I pray that they never have to try like this*.

"*It could have been worse – you might have died*." In the darkest moments of "recovery" this was not the "could have been worse" option. Indeed, particularly the earliest times, life, this life, has not felt like the better end of that deal. There are still days, the less than positive days of which there were so many to begin with, when this thought does not leave me easily.

"*Can't you get hearing aids*?" Or, and on a similar note: "*haven't you got your hearing aids in*?" These comments come from those who just haven't absorbed the reason and nature of my hearing loss, masked as it is by the volume of the tinnitus. The impatience of people who do not have the tolerance with me being deaf just hurts me, again and again.

Those I don't know well can be excused of course, for being totally unaware of the horrendous storm going on in my ears and the din of the extraneous noises. But to be asked "can't you get hearing aids" by someone, when I have explained so many times over my difficulties with hearing – seriously, I wonder is it my hearing that's the problem, or theirs?

I look out at the stillness of the frost and snow, hearing the persistent raging storm that's in my head, knowing that everyone expects the situation to be the reverse, that my world is still, paused, silent. I don't know which I hate more, the persistence of the noise or the need to explain. I don't know either, which of these is having the more negative effect on my sanity.

#

Whilst we're here, if you have suffered VE or ABI or are supporting someone with their recovery, we'll need more than a few bullet points on the finer details of those polite health exchanges people will (a) want to have with you or (b) feel obliged to have with you when you've been seriously ill and have ABI or similar, ongoing difficulties. The (a) or (b) largely depends on the person and their relationship with you.

In my experience with the VE, health enquiries themselves take three forms – one is very rare and is the typical attitude of one of life's genuinely caring souls, of whom there are surprisingly few; the other two are platitudes you just learn to deal with:

1) "Catherine, how *are* you?" Easy to mistake for one of the platitudes, a few people will ask after your health and will genuinely want to know. They'll have remembered how you were last time they saw you, but they won't measure it for themselves with a gushing "you look so much better than …." Instead, they might ask something which links back to then "how are you feeling since …." This shows that they listen and respect what you say. What's more, they carry on listening. They'll let you tell of your own progress and be (largely) attentive whilst you tell them. Sadly though, there are very few people like this!

2) "*Catherine!* How are you?" I have discovered that from many people, this is a platitude in the first degree, something they are not really interested in hearing the answer to. They either launch into a tirade about what I need to do to overcome the particular difficulty (to which it's hard to get a word in edgewise), or nod sagely but don't respond at all, before moving onto the next subject on their list or, less gallantly, to the next person.

Of these, it's difficult to know which the worst response is. It is a bit like when I share that the

Neurology department say it may take this or that length of time to achieve X or Y ... I'm then questioned as to whether I'm responding to their suggestions, whether I'm going to do my very best to try to achieve better health ... as if I'm not already putting everything I have into it!
To be honest, it's hard remembering the etiquette of such exchanges: many of these people ask after your health to give themselves the platform from which they can then pass on what they know. This is cynical of me, I know, but it happens so often!
Yet I still fall into this trap because once you're no longer in the 'social' setting of work or activities it's easy to forget that asking after someone's health can be just a cursory agenda item to them, like a handshake: it's not something that people expect an answer to. Once you've been so ill, this is hard to spot because you assume your recent illness is why people are asking, why they're interested. Like my many other re-learning curves since the VE, I am in the process of re-learning to recognise the platitude of "how are you?" and give the expected "I'm fine" response, telling them nothing rather than actually telling them everything and then being judged for it.

3) The other platitude side-steps asking me how I am and takes the line of telling me how I am instead, all from glimpsing my superior Emperor's attire. This one is so frustrating, it's hard to remain sensible about it, even if I could remember what sensible is supposed to look like. For instance, some true-life - my life - examples include:

- "Look at you in town! You're doing so well!"

No, today is actually a very crap day but I had to fetch my prescription / go for my acupuncture / get more Tena pads.

- "You're walking much better."

That's because I've now moved onto the fabulously undignified stage of self-catheterising! So, at least I don't have to wear adult nappies around my nethers, which makes it somewhat easier to walk with some level of comfort and a darn-sight less awkwardness.

Now I only have to concentrate on getting my legs to go in the right direction.

- "You're hearing much better"

No, I'm not hearing better, today I'm just managing better. I'm not too anxious today so my tinnitus is not too bad.

Now so, this particular conversation has many variations, especially when it's a phone conversation. All the way along, I've told everyone what I've been told: that my hearing's not going to improve and yes, the aids help to an extent, but they also increase the volume of the tinnitus. Having to re-explain this over the phone is a total frustration. Oh and yes I manage better over the phone because I can put that on loud-speaker. I can't do that with people or at social gatherings, so no, the hearing's not better it's just that some days, some ways are more manageable than others.

- "You speak very well for someone who is deaf"

Well, I haven't always been deaf, so that's fortunate for me, but speaking "very well" requires lots of effort and every word comes from a place of uncertainty.

- "You're remembering everything so well."

Erm, no, I just looked at my list.

- "Aren't you ready yet?"

Let's be clear about this one: after a brain injury, almost every process is slower, so things take time, from thinking and processing to actions. What's needed is plenty of time, not plenty of nagging.

... and so it goes on.

#

Then there are those people who approach with the tell, don't ask method, I have discovered the 'street doctors' as I call them. These unqualified medics offer more opinions than any medic I have ever met and have an infallible belief that they know all the answers. Largely this knowledge is based on the experiences of a friend-of-friend or relative who had something similar. However, as I learned from that other patient who I was put in touch with, the way we are all affected by it varies and I have no wish to compare myself, much less be compared.

#

When talking to someone recovering from VE or indeed other conditions, it's worth remembering the distinct difference between hobbies and therapeutic activities. In a conversation with yet another well-meaning soul, much later on in my recovery, I remark that I don't have a day to call my own "what with the gym and the Nordic Walking ..."

"Ahhh, yes," I'm wistfully told, "but they are leisure, aren't they? I'd love to have the time to do that!"

I'm amazed that people can completely miss the fact that these things are prescribed by my GP or the physio and are to help me get back some muscle tone from all that time I spent regretfully declining. These aren't a choice of "me-time" activities and on the days I do them, I always have to be in bed by 8pm as a result of the exertions, shortening my day and eliminating any preferable "me-time" activities I might have chosen to delight in *for myself*.

But I do join in some of the fun things, don't I? Some people want to remind me of this almost, I think, because they want to paint up the picture of me as "back to normal." Join the dots which make up the whole pattern of the complete person again. I get reminded that when there is something special on I have been able to stay up for it, haven't I? Oh yes, that's right, it's happened about 3 times in the past 18 months and the only reason I can manage to do it at all is knowing I can stay in bed next day. But of course to everyone else, that's considered to be the duvet day treat it isn't, rather than the lying in an exhausted state, waiting for a semblance of recovery, which it is.

#

I suppose any list comprising of what not to say should be tempered with guidance as to those better options. Again though, it's subjective and of course very personal, to say the least. One platitude I've been kind of waiting to hear (deafness puns aside, of course) is this one: "Catherine, I'm so sorry this has happened to you."

This is one of the first things someone says to you when you've been bereaved: you are offered condolences, genuine and sincere. During January, February and March, part of me died. Not with the full-on drama of a resuscitation on a hospital trolley, which no-one can ignore, but with the insidious work of the thief, of Viral Encephalitis or any form of Encephalitis for that matter. No big performance but stealthy destruction of vital neurons, my innate skills and intelligence, the cells of my "self" just killed off by the virus.

No one passes on their condolences for this, just their platitudes which at best can seem well-meaning, yet double up as hurtful, dismissive snipes at this other "self", my bereaved self. And at worst? At worst, acknowledgement of this loss is not offered because it's already been accepted by them, if not you, that this is your lot, your like-it-or-lump-it. And if it hasn't been accepted by you ... then isn't it time it was? Shouldn't you be thinking positive? It could have been worse, you could have had cancer ... you should be grateful, you could have died, you know?

So it seems that no one grieves for the part of me who did die, except me, who remembers her best.

20. Medication vs Condition vs "It's Your Age, Dear"

Of all the difficult adjustments that Viral Encephalitis has created for me, adjusting to being catapulted into a set of on-going symptoms is a real struggle. It's compounded for sure by the fact that the Acquired Brain Injury which should speak for itself (not with a whisper but a roar in my ears) presents itself instead in a form which is so easily dismissed by most others with "it's your age, dear."

This dismissal of everything I have gone through to recover as much of my *self* as possible from the thief has been understandable and intolerable in equal measures across the course of my recovery … and I mean across the *whole* course of it. When I think on it, the drama of my illness has been played out just like one of Shakespeare's most profound tragedies, across three distinct acts:

* Act I: Being so ill with the condition itself.
* Act II: Recovery, which is actually being so sick with both the residual effects of the illness and the medication to treat the on-going symptoms: recovering from the effects of all that is the longest act you could possibly have to sit through.
* Act III: Reaching the plateau, which is apparently the best recovery I can hope to obtain. The me that I have become.

#

Act I: Of course I was only an extra in this Act. The main player was the thief, who had all the best lines and kept the drama going, unfolding it carefully to the unwitting audience of my family and myself, the unknowing performer. At this stage, a poorly rehearsed puppet, I was unaware of my central role. Anything and everything that happens is recorded by the audience and pondered upon as "part of the condition." Finally that condition is identified as Viral Encephalitis and the audience applauds with relief.

#

Act II: That whole "ignorance is bliss" platitude held forth for only so long. By Act II, my situation is all about the medication and its role in my recovery and in particular those steroids. An interesting medication, widely used to treat a whole range of conditions and to aid recovery from many serious illnesses and types of surgery, steroids seem to be the oxymoron of the medicine world: they aid my body's repair, but undermine its behaviour and confuse my already addled mind.

The main problem with taking steroids is that they can completely cloud the effects of the condition. After diagnosis – the condition – comes the medication. From here on, conversations with the physicians are punctuated with the idea that many of the on-going symptoms are now down to the medication. I know it's true to an extent: what used to be impatience or urgency has now become paranoia for even the simplest events. During the highest doses of steroids, this steroid-induced paranoia is indiscernible from the ABI and takes control of most of my days. I'm possessed with an urgency which is almost impossible to contain, I become like a child marking off the dates until Christmas and, worse, I'm cheating, marking off days before they arrive, wanting to get to where I don't even know I'm going, in reality and in my own head.

On being discharged from the hospital, my dose is 60mg of steroids daily. In their quest to get on top of the illness, the steroids turn me into someone I would rather not be, as well as the person the thief has made me … more moron than oxy. I'm paranoid, distressed, upset and unable to be acceptable to anyone, especially myself. The dreams and waking nightmares terrify me and I'm powerless to rationalise them. I'm caught somewhere between logical thinking and the fears of my soul or heart, the images of what was happening don't belong to me, yet only I can see them. I would never hurt anyone but as I've explained before, I see myself responsible for the most hideous of accidents, including, knives, accidents to hands from the bloody juicer, hands getting caught, despite what I know, I *know* about the juicer's safety features. And the worse thing? It just doesn't stop.

Act II, this "it's the medication" stage, has many contributory scenes, many of which are outlined across this book. I'm at centre stage of course but am a co-star to the neurologist whom I look to for my cues. At one stage, towards the end of 2008 when my steroid dose is high and my capacity very low, my hydrotherapist asks me if I'd like to see the neurologist sooner, rather than later. I don't ask her to, but she does have a word with the neurologist and my review appointment is brought forwards.

Sam and Evie pick me up for my appointment and I sit in the car, struggling with the speed of the drive, even about town, clutching my bag with my faithful list in it. As soon as I arrive in the waiting area, I am overwhelmed with emotion. I never really understood how emotion can have such physical responsibilities, yet here, in a waiting room which by now should be familiar and reassuring, I'm shaking, tearful and reactionary. My body is becoming as out of control as my mind and I struggle, really struggle to rationalise why, once again, I'm here. I wait in chairs, checking my list to try to calm myself. I have plenty to be positive about: my list has gone from 32 questions in those early appointments, to about 15.

The neurologist calls me in, once again welcoming but watchful as I struggle into his room and then into the waiting chair. Sam comes in with me, in case I forget to ask something or, as often happens, forget the answers he gives me. As soon as I can I ask my questions, the main ones being about my headaches and the overwhelming tiredness, both of these he thinks are due to still being on the medication. He talks about medication for the headaches and Sam asks him if this should be different to the ordinary Panadol and he says "yes" a neuro type is apparently needed. A medication for a medication. I ask if this will be a permanent medication and he says yes again.

Happily, he reduces the steroids by another 5 mg and, although I know they're prescribed for a purpose, I'm so happy I could hug him. I just feel the sooner I am off these the better. We run through the other questions on my list and, as suspected, the swelling on my neck is again due to the medicine.

My final question is: "can the brain repair itself after Encephalitis?" Really I think I know that the brain does not repair itself, I know from the Encephalitis Society's support materials and from the way I've continued to not be able to tap into resources that I thought I had, to aid my recovery or the parts of myself that appear to have been so misplaced. He reassures me that other parts of the brain can take over, to an extent. Sam asks him about taking a drink over

Christmas and he said yes, so I now ask my question about flying.

"When are you planning on flying?" he asks.

"I'm not," I tell him, "I just want to know." For some reason, like the driving, it seems important to me to know that I have an option. He says it should be ok now.

He is just such a nice man, the only professional in my care who I have met who actually gives me the time I need to go through my list. He always gives me straight answers although he seldom says much. Today though, he suggests acupuncture for the headaches. He is the one person who I believe I would want to talk to if anything went wrong because, even now, full of steroids and talk of much of my situation being down to "the medication" I still have a fear of things going badly wrong again.

It's just as well that I feel secure in his care because I do see him often, for a long time and each time with a list. Towards the end of 2008, my lists still look like this:

1. Ears: the never ending tinnitus, it is enough to drive me insane.
2. Legs and feet: my legs decide not to work at times, becoming excessively cold and stiff when I sit. They're cold to touch even when I get up in the morning and they've been under the duvet. The skin feels tender and sore and my leg muscles are weak. And when they are not cold, they burn, like extremities in the snow. This, and the cold, also affects my mobility … I feel like I'm drunk when I get up in night for bathroom.
3. Memory: it's ok to some extent now, when I am engaged with someone or something, but the minute that connection is gone, there is nothing else unless I've written myself a note, a reminder. But then there's no guarantee I'll remember what my note means once I've put it down – and that's if I even remember where I've put it. And my words … I have lost, forgotten so many words. I feel ignorant at times when I can't find the words I need.
4. Headache: mostly on right side, severe at times.
5. Emotions: I often feel detached or devoid of feelings, when things happen which would have upset me previously. Although this means I'm not so

tearful, it also counts the other way: I have no joy, no sense of fun. Overall though, I think I'm less paranoid / obsessed about things.

Of course it makes little sense discussing this at a neurology appointment where I continue to have the least control over my emotions; not an appointment goes past without my becoming emotional from the moment I arrive in the waiting room until the minute I leave with his additional referrals or prescriptions and extra instructions ringing, literally it feels of course, in my ears. I sit explaining a strange detachment from my emotions with tears coursing down my face, like I don't know what I'm talking about. On the plus side, the neurology department is the one place in the hospital , or indeed outside of it, where you are tolerated for not really knowing what you're talking about!

6. Concentration: poor.

7. Clumsy: I trip over my feet, my balance is not great.

8. Still incontinent + erratic bowel: the details of this are not for the faint-hearted.

9. New GP, having to go over things every time.

10. Tiredness: I have to be in bed by 8 - 9pm and some days it's a struggle to get there. I have no energy or enthusiasm for anything more at the end of the day, by around 7-8 pm.

The neurologist listens patiently to my list. For the incontinence he prescribes antibiotics, for the emotional side he prescribes anti-depressants. Am I depressed? I suppose it would be hard not to be in the circumstances, but if I could just feel better, not feel like this, from the condition, from the medication, from the struggle, wouldn't that be the better thing?

#

By March 2009 I am still very emotional about visits to the neurologist and I'm even more so this time around. These always feel like "big" appointments, but this one even more so, as the steroids have been gradually reducing and last time he hinted that it might be possible to come off them before the summer. I try not to attach too much importance (and emotion) to the chance of this, but I can't help the physical shiver of the ever-ready tears, the minute I book in at the registration desk for my appointment.

My curtailed anticipation is rewarded. The neurologist was very pleased with the results of the latest MRI. He patiently listens to me present my list of current questions, symptoms and on-going ailments, before confirming that although many of the items on this list are the on-going result of the condition, some could still be medicine related. So, finally, over a year after the worst of the Viral Encephalitis, he takes me off the steroids and associated meds which he has prescribed. Delighted is not the word for how I feel and of course I cannot describe it, I just show it with my ready tears and surprised smile.

I guess deep down there are still concerns about the emotional angle though, as he does suggest that I continue to see the clinical psychologist. I'm not sure about this although I'm due a review with her anyway. Her group work ended in December and she said she would see us all individually in 6 - 8 weeks. I must remember to pass on the neurologist's request when I see her.

I leave the appointment feeling lighter somehow. Although I'm still very much under his wing in terms of continued care, the fact that on-going medication is now at an end (at least for this part) fills me with both elation and a surprising fear. It's now up to my poor, broken body to support itself in any on-going repair. And as much as I've hated them, with their vicious side-effects, the support the steroids have been giving me will now stop too. My body is on its own.

Within three days of the appointment I take all of my remaining medication to the chemist for disposal. This feels like such a big step. I suppose, and given the theatrical context of events I suppose there might have been a more dramatic scene like popping every pill from its plastic protection and flushing it ceremoniously down the toilet, but I know this is not an eco-friendly thing to do and besides, I prefer the fact that I never to have to pop another steroid! Instead, I place my bag of left-over potions into the safe hands of the pharmacy assistant. After so many months of our interactions taking place the opposite way around, I catch a twinkle in her eye and feel a virtual hug, a glimmer which reassures me that this is a good thing. A really good thing.

So now the medicine has done its job
(I 'm nearly off the medicine)
40mg down to 10
To the Neuro I go, list still in hand
I read all the points I have made
I highlight the old and concentrate on the new
The reply is also new
"Well it's the condition, you see"
The medicine is now free.

I write this poem when the neurologist first hints that the medication might stop soon and it turns out to be providential. In my steroid-free state I attend my review appointments with him and, with my list in hand, we dance to the same tune only the words are different; now it's no longer the medication "it's the condition", you see.

#

Meanwhile, I am constantly concerned about my sight, which seems to be failing. Since losing my hearing I am hyper sensitive to my vision, it seems crucial to me to have a sense which is performing optimally, as a vital link with life but also to having retained something useful, purposeful.

I buy myself a magnifying glass and increase my bedside lighting. These help at first, particularly the light, but before long it doesn't seem so effective, so I guess that's another retest that will need to be done soon. I will ask the neurologist to refer me back to optometry, so I make a point of adding this to my list for next time.

Next time. There's still always a next time. It's a bit like once the NHS have got hold of you they won't let go. I don't know how I managed without a doctor for 10 years, I'm sure I don't. Now medics are a constant part of my life and thank God for them but, in all honesty, I would like to be finished with them.

#

Act III: With the majority of the medication now finished I rely on my complementary therapies and everyone assumes I am "better". As such, any residual effects are down to that marvellous catch-all: my age.

When I say I don't remember things, people say "we all forget!" I know that, of course I know that from before I had this, it's just that it's so different now. It's like I forget there is anything other than what I am doing now, right now, so I write it down. However, then I forget the list or note, I'm oblivious to the post-it or slip of paper until I find it in amongst my piles of paper weeks later. On a good day I might merely stare at it and wonder why I wrote it, or what it's about. On a bad day, I won't even have a glimmer of recall about writing it. I'd think someone else wrote it, I'm that detached from it.

#

People constantly want to compare my incapacity with that of what happens as we age and I resent that. I did not get the opportunity to age gracefully, to adjust. What happened to me happened so fast, there was no gradual aging process, like a carpet gradually wearing away over time. It was more like a rug being pulled out from under. Done. Gone.

#

And the best of me now? Any ache or pain, any and all residual symptoms, the on-going inconvenience of catheterisation, deafness and forgetfulness all play beautifully to an audience, my heart-rending soliloquies about the clock that stopped for me, for the woman I was. Unfortunately, these draw less of a dramatic Shakespearean and more of a pantomime response from the audience ... the prime of my life? "It's behind you".

The trouble is, I wasn't this bundle of symptoms which suggest a woman of a certain age until the Thief in the Night crept up on me. I was always younger than this woman, I'd successfully by-passed being my own age and was cheerfully moving into today's "Third Age" generation of the lively retired, the purposeful, travelling, creative, attentive kind. Instead, I now play the role of a much older woman, until such a time as the curtain drops on this act and I make my last curtain call. OK, I am grateful for the chance of an encore, one which at times I never even believed I would have the energy, much less would have wanted or retained the spirit to make, yet it's a role I find extremely hard to play. This is not my age, dear, it's really not.

21. So This Is The New "Normal"?

It's October but as far as I'm concerned when the clock hands moved from one month into the next, in those wee small hours, it was a bad start to the month. Once again I'm caught up in dreams of rats and mice. I see them playing amongst my birthday cards on the side table, one little one and another, much larger. This larger one looks more like a cartoon character with an emblem on his front as he stands on his hind legs, but he's not amusing like a cartoon character, he's menacing.

I don't know if this is anything to do with the albino squirrel we saw in the park a few weeks ago or because I've not been taking my sleeping tablets this week. I put them out, ready to take them, on two nights running but then fell asleep without them. So I've just carried on without. But now the mice are back.

#

Despite the rigours of night-time again, my days are set to be more cheerful! Well, for today at least, because I'm going on a happiness course. The venue seems OK and there are quite a few people here, who all seem friendly and smiley enough, which I suppose is right given the context of the event.

The trouble is, I'm starting to find it a bit emotional. Happiness, it seems, is as much a trigger for other emotions as itself. Yes, I can go with the happiness vibe, but that doesn't remove that it's so difficult to be part of something this significant, so wordy and poignant, yet to hardly be able to hear any of it. Of course, I'm the only one who really knows I'm not part of it as not everyone knows I'm deaf, which kind of adds to that sense of isolation which comes alongside the hearing loss anyway.

However, there's also another context to the event and I think this too is bombarding me emotionally in a way that I hadn't really predicted, if I'm honest. As counsellors we are obliged to attend three workshops each year, to fulfil the requirements of our continued professional development (CPD) and I've really felt that participating on this one would be a marker for me as the day I got sick was the 26th January, at that first of this triplet of training courses, the CBT training. Today's one, this happiness course, is the last training event of the year, so I'm thinking that it might be a good one to do, a signpost of coming to the end of a year which has been so very extreme. Sometimes I still feel so awful, yet at other times I think I must be getting better as I give priority to external events in life, a bit like this one. There are times when I just want to lie down and rest but instead I push myself on to do a few more chores that need to be done, rather than have them pile up. Always pushing myself, physically, emotionally, trying to get that balance, get back to normal.

So, today's about happiness on the outside but on the inside its about effort and endeavour and being as normal as I can possibly be so that I can come full circle at least in finishing what I started with the training, even though my counselling job is now lost to me. I know deep down that I'm also pushing for this day to be a marker for the illness: it's where it started so this is where it must stop. To that end I am successful, in that I survive the day and, somehow, I manage to get home although I'm so weary I can't really say how I manage it.

I'm also cold, right into my bones. I text Sam to share that I made it through the day, but that I'm very cold and tired and of course the texting takes an age as my numb, frozen fingers jab away at the tiny phone keypad.

I'm just thinking that I don't really even have the energy to think about food, when there she is, my child, coming through the door with fresh spaghetti for me. I can't help it, I just dissolve, sobbing about my state, about my day, about the fact that it's all too bloody much.

#

It's now 7pm and Sam's gone. I'm tucked up in bed, legs aching, feet burning and just needing to lie down and stay there, nothing to do but reflect on my first day of being back to 'normal.'

#

It's Sunday and I'm trying to be up and at it, ready for Mass, although the weather outside is particularly shocking – torrents of relentless, shivering rain. Sam texts me to say she'll take me, but when she arrives she's on her own. It's too wet to bring Evie out, she tells me, so she's coming to Mass too.

It's pleasant coming down here together, companionable. Afterwards, Sam invites me back for a cup of tea so of course I come back with her, to spend a little more time with her and Simon and of course to see my precious munchkin, Evie.

My next mission for the day is to pop into town to get some birthday gifts I need for Monday. Thankfully the weather's dried up considerably, so they all join me. The shopping doesn't take long and on the way back, Sam invites me to come back to theirs later, for dinner and to stay. I know I'm being hesitant because this is unexpected, which of course immediately panics me, but I accept for both activities.

They drop me back home so that I can organise myself with tablets for this evening and herbs for tomorrow morning. I make a list of clothes I'll need, plus lists of things to do like close the curtains, put the lights off, leave a security light on. When I've exhausted my list-making to remove some of that initial stress, I sit down on the bed and allow myself a few moments grace with the other source of my panic: I've been afraid of doing this.

I haven't stayed with them since I moved home in July and I'm afraid, very much afraid of that slippery slope if I stay there. Is staying over a signal of wariness about my independence? Will I be able to come back to my own house? Will the baby nightmares start again? I'm helpless over this situation, it's something that I have to do in order to, once again, gain back some semblance of my old "normal" life. Except it doesn't feel normal, this terror of what came before.

#

We have a grand evening, a lovely roast dinner, an excellent splashing, bubbly fun bathing of the baby session and then game of Scrabble. I take my tablets before sleeping and I do, in a manner of speaking, sleep.

#

A game of Scrabble, yes, there's a thing, wrapped up closely with my writing. My focus and my spelling are mis-matched beyond belief. I still find that if I try to write after a busy day it all goes wrong – I just seem to lose the ability, plain and simple. I know what I want to write but that's not what appears on the paper. I'm not sure where it goes, but my head and hand are not coordinated.

Words also disappear on me. I've been trying to type up a poem I've written and I type 'Buty' – it looks OK but the strict red line of the Windows' spell check keeps telling me it's not correct. I look at it for what seems like an age. I can't see what's wrong with it. Stupid old spell-check, stupid old Microsoft. However, the distraction of the wavy red line beneath my word cannot be underestimated, much less ignored. I'm looking at it with an increasing furrow in my brow and curses on my tongue, for about an hour before the penny drops. The word I need, the title of my poem is Beauty and yet for all this time 'Buty' has seemed OK to me. This isn't the first time this has happened either, it's happened so many times I could probably write a book, but then no-one would understand it because the spelling would be that bad! Spelling was never one of my best subjects but now at times it's like I write a different language.

#

I'm out and about with Sam today. We've had coffee at hers and I've played with Evie whilst she got on with chores, but as soon as we get into the car to follow up our plans, I find my throat bulging with unreleased sobs, whilst tears begin to trickle their usual path down my cheeks.

"I'm just sick of it all," I wail. "I just want to be better."

Sam tells me I am better and I know that's true, to a given extent, but I still don't *feel* like the me I used to be, so I share this. Sam replies that there's nothing that I used to do that I can't do now, but my tears show that I don't agree with her.

Fair play to her, to an extent she's probably right but her comment misses the point that those things I can do, I mostly can't do it independently. Take the incontinence – in fact, yes please, do take the bloody incontinence. There was a time when I could choose the timing of my bodily functions, but now? Can't do that now, I rely on pads, hideously uncomfortable and scarily expensive pads. I used to sing in choral groups, be one of the voices, express myself freely and tunefully through the wonder of song, the joy of music, but now? Can't do that now, I can't hear the music, can't hear to keep the timing, can't hear my own voice to stay in tune – I probably sing with the same tunefulness as the baby seagulls who squawk all spring and summer long around here. So no, I don't agree that I can do everything I used to, not at all.

Sam asks if I want to go home, but I rally myself, as I have lots of shopping to do and there's no point in this, these tears, these comparisons. I have another reality now and within this reality I still need to shop and eat.

Today though, the shopping seems to take me ages because this is a list I've written randomly, as the items have popped into my head or I've used up the last of something. As I shop directly from the list I have to walk the aisles in no particular order to try to find things. I try to use some logic to find them but even so, they're usually not where I think they should be, which frustrates and tires me even more.

I'm having a hard day, it's true, so I do something I wouldn't dream of normally. I find myself in the prepared foods section and I pick up a readymade cottage pie. That'll do for tea, that'll do for me.

Back home, alone, after a rest and a few gentle chores, I eat the pie. Or rather, I get through the pie ... there's no eating with relish or enthusiasm because it's really not the kind of cuisine to be enthusiastic over. Its look not only resembles the bland image on the packaging, but its taste pretty much resembles packaging too, cardboardly chewy, with its own puddle of brightly coloured grease. It's unpleasant to say the least, with an aftertaste which not only lingers in my mouth, behind my teeth, but also comes back to haunt by repeating on me throughout the evening.

So much for feeling sorry for myself and taking an easy route to goodness knows what! Tomorrow it's back to my juicing, my clean diet of home-made food and absolutely no additives.

#

I am at home today because I have another meeting with the social worker lady who deals with putting carers in place. As meetings with professionals go, this one is proving to be another classic.

As it stands, I've been allocated two hours, two days a week, so this social worker has come to tell me which two days I will be given these two hours they deem necessary: one hour housework, one hour shopping. Even without shopping, driving to the supermarket and back would take 20 minutes alone and although I know that anything's better than nothing, I dread to think what kind of housework could be achieved in just one hour.

I ask about the costs for the service. She can't tell me what the charges are exactly but does an approximation which astounds me. I have Carol of course, who helps me from time to time and basically the figure the woman trots off is double what I pay privately, on an ad-hoc basis (and no, it doesn't mean I'm a skinflint where that's concerned, I'm mindful of the going rate and I highly value those who help me and reflect that value in my payments) but this figure she quotes me is just extortionate!

Still, money aside, although she's being sympathetic and friendly and altogether much nicer than she has been (if a little bit patronising), it doesn't take long for us to realise that there's a bigger problem. With my hydro twice a week and various other medical appointments, plus work until the business is sold, she can't slot me in to her programme. It's not flexible, their system, you see. These two hour appointments can not be changed once they are set up but the problem is that Hydro can change every week, doctor's appointments change and of course all the other things I do have to be flexible, even though this in itself is something that I struggle with.

It strikes me as so strange that the people who purport to help you get back to full health are so inflexible themselves, especially as they know that patients like me are so much in the hands of what often proves to be a very chop-and-change medical system. So, the upshot? She decides to put my needs "on hold" for now. She says she'll contact the social worker and tell her, then she takes her leave. So thank God, actually, that that's the end of that, it really does seem that I'm better off in all ways just doing what I'm doing, with Carol's trusted assistance.

#

Hot on the heels of being put "on hold" for a care package, I've received a third letter from the auspicious Department of Work and Pensions today. I have to say I regard the tell-tale envelope with certain suspicion before I actually open it but, here we go.

They write to inform me that I will not qualify for DLA (Disability Living Allowance), because I can walk 100ft, attend to my own personal care (wash myself and of course attend "independently" to the awful incontinence issues), oh and I'm capable of cooking myself a meal. There's nothing about the difficulties of bathing and showering (and I'm sure even a chimp would make a connection with the incontinence here), or the daily problems of being faced with endless household chores that I just can't manage. No, I have it here in black and white, I could be living in a filthy house for want of being able to do things but the fact I can walk a very limited distance makes it all ok.

#

There has been a phone call from the sensory team. My phone is flashing to alert me to the fact there's a message. Erm, let's look at the facts here: a message; on the answer phone; from the sensory people; about the system pertaining to my hearing loss. I have to laugh, seriously I have to laugh, roughly for about as long as it would have taken me to actually hear the message. So, these are the people dealing with my deaf aids but of course I can't hear the message so have to wait until a friend pops in so that she can listen to it for me.

She tells me they say they will be coming on Friday to check the system as it has been reported not working correctly. OK, that was a whole month ago, so which Friday are we talking about here? It's strange that the people who should know (in fact I'm being charitable there, they *do* know) how difficult the phone is for me, do tend to still phone me as the primary means of contact, because it's convenient *for them*.

This includes the social worker, whom I have met twice but apparently have missed lots of calls from. Co-incidentally she calls this afternoon, to say she has had a call from her Head of Care. It seems that, contrary to what I was told the other day, my case will now be closed as they can't put cases on hold. It doesn't mean I don't need help of course, it just means that they won't help me.

#

The month slowly moves on. Today sees Sam, Simon and Evie go off to France for a long weekend, they won't be back until late Monday, I think. They text me to let me know that they called by with paper for me this morning, but I didn't hear the doorbell via the pager, nor feel the vibrator pad which is supposed to alert me, this being the system which is not working properly. So I missed them, didn't get to wish them "bon voyage" something which upsets me, incredibly so.

#

It's Monday and I'm just home as my hydro is now twice a week: Monday and Thursday. When I don't have a lift or need to get a cab due to other appointments, I still persist with the lurking by the window routine which goes with waiting for the hospital transport, like today.

To kill the time I've made a list of things to do, I phone the DVLA to check if I need to report my deafness to them before I get back into the driving seat. As far as I can make out, the woman says that's not necessary, unless I'm a bus or lorry driver. This feels like really good news for me and I hug the idea to myself whilst I carry on waiting for the transport. It actually feels more real, more exciting than when I got the letter to say, in beautifully formal-speak, that "following medical investigation for Encephalitis" I could now drive. I suspect the way I feel isn't so much to do with the news itself and more to do with my own confidence issues: I feel much nearer to being ready to drive, although of course I still haven't tried. However, it does seem like such good news that I then doubt myself and wonder if I heard her properly, so when Sam and Simon get back, I'll ask them to call and check for me, to be on the safe side and, joy of joys, when Simon phones for me, they give him the same answer.

#

As the month moves on, I'm feeling a little stronger and find that I'm able to do a bit more without all the pain ... it's still there mind, but not so severe. Today is a work day and I'm up early, although somewhat too early. I find myself with an hour to spare before Ron's due to pick me up to take me to the office.

As I aimlessly tidy bits and pieces around the bedroom, my eye falls to my wardrobes. Now there's a job that's been bothering me for some time, so I decide to tackle them. You'd not believe the mess they're in, there's evidence of their abandonment in January, with clothes I bought in the January sales still bearing their price tags and of course unworn because of the steroid balloon I became shortly afterwards. I'm still aware of the need to pace myself, so I start by putting away all my summer clothes. However, starting is one thing, getting the task finished is quite a different thing entirely but for today at least, start is what I do. I hump a case onto the bed for the summer bits, and open up a black bag, ready for the charity shop and I quietly potter, ponder and fold until Ron arrives.

#

It's Monday again. Once I'm eventually dried and dressed, the physiotherapist says that she thinks I'm getting a bit stronger, so she's suggesting we set goals on our Monday sessions, for me to aim for during the week.

I don't hesitate. I tell her that for this week finishing the relentless sorting out of the wardrobe will be my goal. In truth, I think she meant a physical exercise, but I know how doing this job alone gives me lots of exercise, so she agrees to it.

"How is your sight?" she then asks.

Part of me wonders why she's asking, what she's noticed, but another part of me shouts down the paranoia and I answer her honestly. I tell her that I do think it's deteriorated, although back in March ophthalmology said there was no significant change in my prescription. Now though, I feel there is and I tell her, quite openly about my difficulty with reading from both the sight and concentration aspects.

Her expression says it all and she admits that she's surprised to hear that I have difficulty with reading, because I'm so articulate in my conversations with her and she never imagined that reading would be any different from speech. I'm supposing too that the same applies to my hearing, because I'm seen to be managing, I must be managing, mustn't I? So there we are, another case of my Emperor's new clothes, or should that be spectacles?

I sometimes wonder if others could imagine how it feels to be in a situation such as I am. They can have no idea, not really. They all say, "you look well, you walk well." But again it's about what they can't see that really bothers me, not that I want them to see the incontinence of course, perish the thought, but you understand my meaning. So it all goes on, all these hidden extras that the thief left behind, including this constant noise in my ears on top of which people shout when then know I can't hear them, yet that never helps - clarity is what is needed, in all aspects.

#

It's Friday and I am feeling very satisfied with myself. My wardrobes are finished, I've met my goal. In all, this has been a good week, I've felt more like myself again at times; my walking has improved, my emotions have felt more in balance and I guess I've just felt more able in general. I've just realised that in fact I've taken on more and achieved more. Yes, it's been a good week.

#

I'm having another week of being busy, doing more myself, trying to be more myself. Last week I phoned the doctors a few times for an appointment but have to fall in with their system of only being allowed to book the appointment on the day, rather than in advance. So, I tackle that one first thing today, Monday and am offered one for this afternoon, which is good news. The bad news? This is the GP I'd rather not see. They're a husband and wife team and I usually see her husband who is gentle in his approach, but today I can only see his wife who I find very abrupt and sharp.

So, I make sure I prepare with my list of all my symptoms and queries, to help ensure I don't get disconcerted by the doctor and forget anything.

The outcome of my list broadly reflects the quality and quantity of time I spend at the appointment:

1) A heavy discharge – to which she says, "we'll take a swab".

2) A pain in my left breast – "it's muscle" she says, without checking me. I tell her we've checked this before so she returns to her notes, constantly repeating "no ... no." I then tell her "yes, my daughter was with me ... you examined me in front of her, I remember because of this, because it was so embarrassing." This, a disturbing, poignant

memory for me means nothing to her. She points again to her notes, "nothing here."

3) Sore throat and sore lips – she looks at my throat. "nothing" she says.

4) I am losing a lot of hair, it's falling out – response: "nothing we can do about that."

5) Constant headaches – part of the condition.

6) Sleeping tablets, I tell her I am cutting them out at times.

She asks, "so you cut and take half?"

"No," I reply, "I just don't take them some nights."

I'm little the wiser when I come out; it just feels like a huge waste of time going to see her.

#

I have a phone call this week to say Emer my niece has given birth to a baby girl. It makes me think about my family and my context within my family. The occasional phone calls and expectance of gratitude each time is wearing; some call me once a week or text me, which is grand, but I feel as though all my brothers but one have disappeared.

My paranoid self, still touched by the thief, suggests that this is the price I have to pay for long-term illness, the fact I've just dropped off others' radar. But then I think, well that's just daft talking … the truth is nothing's really changed; my brothers didn't keep in touch with me before, so it is no different now, is it? The question of whether it *should* be different now though, is another one altogether.

#

My busy week took an unexpected turn this morning, in a way which I've not only adapted to, but am extremely happy about. Evie is now with me for a few hours this morning. She can't go to nursery because she was sick yesterday and of course, with infection control being a very necessary thing for these little ones, she has to stay away from nursery and have 24 hours clear of vomiting. The thing is though, she's not sick in that sense just snotty, bless her, and when she has mucus it always makes her vomit.

So Evie and I get to spend the morning being a grandmother and a granddaughter together. Yes, I still fear for her but don't want to let the paranoid weight of this precious responsibility pin me down with fear, I want to be able and I want to be here for her. So, for this morning at least I ignore the fears the same as I ignore the rats and ghouls and I wrap myself in the warm delight of my granddaughter.

#

Following our successful babysitting session, Sam's asked me to babysit Evie on my own this evening at their house, and sleep over. This is my very first time of having Evie at night and the thought terrifies me, with prospects too awful, too fearful to ponder.

Even fanciful fears aside, my practical limitations are also a concern. My hearing, or indeed lack of it, makes it difficult: I cannot hear her on the monitor, so if she's in her cot I need to stay upstairs. I broach this concern with Sam and she agrees that it's better for me if I let her sleep downstairs, perhaps laying her on the couch once she drops off.

So that's the plan, although of course the delightful minx has other ideas. Having given her the bedtime bottle and cuddled her whilst she wriggled about, we then look at her books together until, eventually she falls asleep about an hour later than usual. Of course she's a good girl, but tonight she's certainly restless.

Now she's settled I realise how stiff I have become and of course so very tired as it's practically my bedtime too! I stand up to have a stretch. It's no good, I need to walk it off a bit and I could do with some water too. I make my way to the kitchen to get my drink but, as I walk back into the living room I see my poppet turning over in her sleep. The moment is caught in slow motion as she turns and for a second it looks as if she's just going to get off the couch but of course she's asleep and instead she slides, gracefully assisted by her fleecy sleepsuit against the leather of the couch, off the sofa.

My heart's in my mouth. In a heart-beat it's over and I haven't had time, despite my efforts, to dash over, to catch her. Instead, she slips, still dreamlike, onto a cushion on the floor where she immediately puts her head down to sleep again.

She's sleeping peacefully whilst I'm broken, absolutely broken. After all the months of worries about if I hurt her, if I let her fall, fell with her in my arms, oh the thought of it is just awful ... these waking nightmares, they've never gone away and now one is real. For a while they've been infrequent but they're still here and tonight they're back with a taunting vengeance.

I sit for a long while, terrified to move, just watching the gentle rise and fall of her chest, the flicker of her eyelids, the pucker and dribble of her little lips. At some point, reason starts to stave off the fears and the thought pops into my head that it's going to be a long night indeed if this is all I do for the duration. So, finally I move myself and gingerly set up the ironing, which I manage to do without burning myself, something of a miracle seeing as I do not take my eyes off the baby throughout.

Sam and Simon aren't late, it wasn't a riotous night out, just a local pub quiz. We have a cup of tea and go to bed calm and happy that the evening was a success.

Or so it would seem. Truth be told, the stress and adrenalin are still running through me, I can't stop seeing Evie sliding off the sofa. I don't really understand why I am trusted with this child, when I am trusted with so little else and now I've shown that I can't even do that. It's now 1.20 am and I'm back downstairs, getting the water I need to take the sleeping tablet I'm finally succumbing to. Back upstairs again I wait for it to work, but it's a long time coming. I lay here watching my own fears dancing in front of me, until work worries take over instead, when will I do this, have I done that yet? Right in front of me I see Antony fall off the ladder and hurt himself, kind Antony who helps me, runs around for me, helped me when I lost my phone ... I lay here imagining these awful things and I can't switch it off, this horrific vein of thinking just does not stop and it's not really nice things, not nice things at all.

#

For the last few days I've stayed at home. No matter what lifts are offered, I can't get in a car, much less get a train or a bus and go somewhere. My confidence and physical strength have deserted me, so now my weekly aims are right back to square one, to once again get these back. It's a long, slow slog and I'm so very tired of it.

Sam's dropped by on her way home from work with a lovely bunch of lilies for me. I've shown real pleasure in them for her sake, I've arranged them in a vase and put them somewhere I'll enjoy them. Trouble is, try as I might to bring this to mind as something nice, it's just not working. I seem to be back in that other place.

#

So I'm trying very hard to get back to the other "normal" that I had just weeks ago. Today is a pretty good one in that respect. Sam's helped me to make beds up and hoover the two top rooms as Ann and Robert will be coming on Sunday and staying the night. The following weekend my sister comes again, so there will be plenty of distractions.

Once Sam's left for her beautician's appointment, I hoover the living room myself then wash the kitchen floor. Now I'm like some dippy woman from a TV ad, standing to admire my shiny floor because this is another achievement for me – my first floor wash, without the machine, since July when I came home. I spend a good few minutes admiring the floor, then another few recovering both my strength and my sensibilities!

Sam pops back, the plan is that she'll drop me off at the supermarket on her way home. I'm relieved to see her return as promised and realise that I haven't actually been anxious about it this time around ... another major breakthrough! Having and being able to display this trust is a major improvement for me; the fact that Sam or whoever can say they'll be back in an hour, I can trust in that and manage the anxiety much better now. It's a relief, such a relief, not to be constantly at the window, waiting.

And so, once she's back it's off to the supermarket. I have my lists and I have nothing to rush about for, so I find myself taking my time, happily leaning on my trolley, not just rushing from A to B according to my list but also taking a little time to mooch. This way, I've managed to do both my food shopping and make a start on some of my Christmas shopping. I fold myself into a taxi to come home and I'm glad to be here.

#

I'm using my stick less and less as my joints are less painful. For some reason, after all these months of clean diet and juicing, my energy seems to be taking an upturn. I don't know what this shift is due to but I'm trying to make the most of it. Actually, I think it may have a little to do with acceptance. I am deaf, I can't change that and, somewhere along the line I seem to have accepted it. I am stiff and sore but I don't have to accept that, I can work on it and so I do. That's true of many things in fact, anything that I can work on, I do and I guess, like my light-bulb moment of finding I had to be a *patient* patient, it's been the getting to this point of acceptance which is most helpful to my overall physical and emotional recovery.

#

I'm having a crisis – I've just received a letter from Hastings and Rother Counselling Service to say that there's another workshop on 22nd November on Emotional Freedom Techniques (EFT). I'm sure I've already got something on then and it seems such short notice ... I really don't know what to do. It takes me a good few moments, of staring anxiously at the letter to realise that although I think 22nd November is next week, it is in fact a whole month away! Oh how easy it is for a crisis to appear to loom, but then be knocked aside by a moment's blissful clarity. I'm too relieved to be upset with myself for getting in a tizz so, here I am, cutting myself a bit of slack!

#

There are other indicators that I am getting better, subtle, but definitely there. When I see a spot of dirt or clutter that annoys me, I try to do it myself rather than wait until I have a willing helper. Like my wardrobes and like this, my bedside collection of plugs and wires, medications and creams, oh gosh yes, I'm so fed up with the clutter of medication and creams. I play around with the arrangements, moving my lamp to the other side of the bed. OK, so the medicines and potions must stay for now, but I have reduced the clutter a bit.

#

It's almost the end of the month so I stick with an age-old habit and start on my Christmas cards. It's not usually a chore for me, more something that I enjoy and I like to be organized so I want to give myself plenty of time to do it and, in the context of my writing, do it properly. My plan is that I intend to do a few every morning and so I've laid them out in the study with the address labels already printed.

It takes a bit of time for me to realise that although my writing seems good enough, even good in general to start with, when I try to do too much, for too long, it goes again. This morning, I've been killing time whilst waiting for the hydro transport, so I've stayed at it far longer than the 30 minutes I usually aim to spend. By the end of it, I realise that my writing is appalling, like a child's graffiti instead of my loving, heartfelt greeting for the season.

I find myself getting upset, not just for the quality of my writing or for my own failure once again to pace myself appropriately but for the cold, bold truth that this time last year this job would have taken me just a few nights and I'd have enjoyed it, not slogged through it.

It doesn't help that my headaches have been so bad again, these last few days and I'm still so very tired. I can't stand this combination, this overwhelming tiredness I remember so well and cope with pretty much constantly, but when it comes with the headaches too, I'm gripped with the fear that it's all coming back again, that something's wrong. All these individual pains, headaches, tiredness, I appreciate that they all sound simple enough, but it's having them all going on at the same time that wears me down.

I relate this tale of woe to the physio when I get to hydro. For her part, she thinks I've got stronger and that the time's now right to go back to one session each week. She asks me if I feel like I am going backwards and, despite trying to always look at the positives, I answer a plain and simple "yes." She then says that she could have a word with the neurologist for me if I'd like and I know that my eyes are bright, tearful bright as, once again, I give my plain and simple "yes."

#

It's Hallowe'en and the trick or treat of the day is that I'm at work. Ron's helping out and we're very busy but it's satisfying ... I finally feel like I'm doing my job some days. My head's a little better but I'm so cold. That's not just me though ... the weather has really turned, bitterly cold with snow in some parts of the country. The clocks have gone back too, so darkness and all its demons arrive by 5pm, so I make sure I'm home well before then.

And speaking of demons of course, as it's Hallowe'en I prepared for callers. I buy chocolate eye sweets and bats, which all lie in a bowl ready to be shared with excited, ruddy cheeked or face-painted trick or treaters.

However, after much preparation and anticipation on my part, the first ring of the doorbell for the evening finds me rooted to the spot, mortally afraid to answer the door. This feeling of being involved is important, so very important after everything, yet to find myself so completely unable to action this involvement is both ridiculous and mortifying in equal measures. This inaction of mine, this failure to fulfil the treat end of the bargain brings tricks worse than any Hallowe'en revellers could inflict on me. My guts wrench with the familiar fear: with the headaches, pains and aches, I'm terrified it will go wrong again and that something bad is brewing. How can I cope with this conflict, hanging on to shreds of positivity about a full recovery whilst being bombarded with flashes of what might be looming?

Amongst it all, the physio phones, to say that my neurologist has agreed to try to bring my December appointment forward to the next couple of weeks.

22. The Sound of Silence (It's Louder Than You'd Think)

When I move back home, in July 2008, it suddenly becomes very important, very necessary that I have the right equipment to meet my hearing needs. Clearly what we've been doing at Sam's is muddling through the situation but now, home alone and deaf to the world, I'm vulnerable in a whole new way.

Sam makes some phone calls to a social worker to ask how we to go about getting some hearing equipment. The social worker advises us to go over to Eastbourne, where a hearing charity run a voluntary set up, which has all the equipment that someone with my hearing problems would want to try. She advises us that this is the best course of action, particularly in terms of my need for a phone – both for emergencies and contact with the outside world as, according to her, waiting for the wheels of "the system" to turn would take weeks.

So Sam takes me to Eastbourne. It turns out not to be the quick and simple task we had hoped. We spend three hours of trials with different equipment and appliances, before we establish that a loop system for the TV would be compatible with my hearing aids.

The choice for the phone comes down to two options: one a base unit with two extra receivers, all hands free, made by Panasonic; the other a big button phone with volume and tone control, which can be used hands-free at the touch of a button. Although I like this phone because I can hear best from it, it has the huge disadvantage of being so old-fashioned. Of course, I'm not that worried about it looking dated, but it's the fact that it's a corded phone and it doesn't come with two handsets. With my difficulties with mobility, the benefits of the other phone having a handset I can keep upstairs with another kept downstairs seems to give it a distinct advantage even though the sound quality is not so good for my particular hearing difficulties.

I find the decision making process difficult and am so grateful to have Sam's company, both to remind me about my own questions and to ask things I wouldn't even have thought of. There is so much to take in and even when they ask me questions about my own disabilities, I find it hard to remember the answers, which sounds like madness but I guess is proof of the ABI itself, as if it were needed. It's good of them not to rush us over the decision-making, which I still find very stressful. Our three hour stint there is testament to the volunteers' helpful, patient natures and they offer only help, not pressure with my decision. Finally, my indecisiveness and overwhelming tiredness leads to a decision of sorts: I buy the old fashioned one so that I can hear *and* the Panasonic with its three handsets, to allow me to answer and gain time to get to the one that I can hear through!

#

Within a month of my returning home, to my home, my son Simon comes to stay. This time around is the first time we've seen each other since my hearing has deteriorated so significantly and I don't know which of us it appears more markedly to. It's lovely to see him and be at home with him, sitting companionably and having good dinners together, but the chat is of course not free flowing. I can't hear him properly and it's so difficult for him to get used to the need to look at me when he speaks.

There's frustration in repetition too, of course: I find it as incredibly frustrating to have to repeat several times to him "what did you say?" or "I didn't hear that" as he does to have to continually repeat himself. We manage, after a fashion, to sit and do the crossword but mostly we just spend time sitting in companionable silence, broken with gentle chat. This is the best I can do just now.

#

My next hospital appointment at the ENT department at the hospital comes soon after this. Thankfully I see the same doctor that I saw last time. It sounds like a small thing, but this is something I have learned to be grateful for, as it's exhausting seeing new faces and having to explain and re-explain the reasons why I've been referred, why I'm sitting in front of them. I tell him the tinnitus has got worse so he sends me across the hall to have another hearing test. As he puts the headphones on me, he tells me there will be a whooshing noise and that if it gets too much I should just keep my finger on the buzzer and he will then switch it off. It doesn't get too much, I just sit there, waiting and hoping for something extraordinary to happen.

When he has finished I tell him the constant noise in my ears from the tinnitus is worse than the noise in the test. He just says "nice" in a voice which gives nothing away. We then have a chat for a few minutes and he tells me I will need to go back to the doctor's office and that he's going to suggest that I go to see someone else. So, off I go back to the waiting area whilst my doctor sees the consultant, before I am called in. He tells me that I have lost 10 - 20 decibels in my left ear and that if I can get to London again he wants to refer me to a hearing therapist. He says that she is a doctor in St George's Hospital in Tooting, but he would like me to have blood tests first. I ask again if this issue with my hearing is from the condition or is drug induced, from the medication. He is not sure, but seems to think it's more likely that it is an auto immune issue, as this showed in previous blood tests. As this has been a long appointment, the Pathology Department is now closed, so it'll be tomorrow for the blood tests.

So I go back the next day, for another round with the medical vampires. It doesn't take too long, but leaves me very bruised; my poor veins just don't seem to want to play these games any more. I also come away with a very mixed sense of disappointment tinged with relief: disappointment that they're now thinking that it's due to something else, having said for so long previously that it was all due to the drugs necessary to fight the virus. This is tempered only by the relief that knowing another referral is being made. The hospital they've mentioned, St. George's, is just a few miles from where I used to live in London. I feel a strange sense of going back, but yet again as another person entirely.

#

As my hearing-set up at home improves, a man comes to fit the smoke alarms, the door bell, phone sensors and loop system for the TV. Now I have to carry a pager to tell me that the phone or door are ringing or, worse, to alert me if the smoke alarms are frantically trying to tell me that the house is on fire!

I feel a bit like an infant with name tag, a toy, a raggie ... some prized possession that I must clutch at all times. The difference is that for an infant someone else carries them, looks out to make sure they've got them or haven't lost them. I have only myself and my notes to remind me to use these things and, even when I remember to use them, by the time these sensors have relayed their relevant messages, my mobility is such that I can only respond with a certain (OK, minimal) level of agility; being alert to the fact that someone's trying to contact me doesn't help me to get to the door or phone any faster. In truth, I'm still missing as many calls and callers as I did before having these useful extras and have the extra dissatisfaction of both being attached to items "for my own safety", just like having that awful purse around my neck with the mobile in it during those early "home alone" days at Sam's house, along with now knowing that I've missed out on a visitor or a call. When I think about this, it feels like I have made no progress at all.

#

When I'm alone, in my own home, I am often caught unawares by an absolute grief for my hearing loss, followed with an overwhelming sense of isolation and exclusion. I've begun to realise that being deaf ends impromptu conversation and plunges you into a very lonely and detached place.

When I tell a friend that I feel I'm missing out on so much she asks, sympathetically "what do you miss?" It's one of these questions which inspires an outpouring, a list I haven't written but have clearly been bottling, brooding and building up for some time. I take her politely-offered enquiry and run with it, readily rattling off what is missing from the auditory circle of my life, as I now know it:

> * Talking on the phone: sure, I know I've got an adapted phone at home now, but it's not the same. There's the phone at work that I can't just pick up and use to run my business, re-establish myself at the helm of my own life because the phone at my office desk quite simply never rings. It's constantly diverted to someone out of the office, someone who can hear it ring, answer it and hold a sensible exchange with the person on the other end. A person who isn't me, the owner of the company. I've been outsourced.

* Music: both listening to it in the background of my home and events, as well as being a part of it, with the singing group that I belonged to. This is a gap in my life I cannot contemplate for too long without becoming terribly emotional, still. There is nothing tuneful or melodic about the noise in my ears, it's not even the anticipatory warming up notes of the band about to get started, it's just noise.
* Theatre: both the performance and the social side of going to the theatre, the participation of appreciation in the performance, the fun critique or compliment of the quality of the show, the acting, dancing, singing or whatever. This is now alien to me. As I'm sure I've said before, the price of the ticket is just wasted on me.
* The general chit-chat of get-togethers: whether with family, friends or both - I miss being involved in the deep and meaningful nuances of conversations, of what's *not* being said within the inflections and intonations passed on through what *is* said. I have to focus on the person who is speaking with such intensity that I miss all the other interactions going on around me and even some of those directed to me. In a way, conversations are like my experiences with reading now: I am so caught up in the mechanics that half the time I miss the meaning of what is being conveyed, the actual essence of what is shared.

#

Some days I think I have forgotten what I used to sound like, not just in respect of my singing, which truly makes me sad, but just the sound of me, the voice that is mine. I can't moderate myself and cannot adjust my tone or volume without being reminded that I'm being too loud or too brusque ... yet all I'm really trying to do is be a part of a conversation.

It also saddens me when I think, will I ever know what new people sound like, what little Evie's babbling and earnest communications really sound like to the ears of a first-time Grandma. I know the sounds of a child, of course, but this child ... I don't know her voice at all. I am told she is trying to say "grandma". How I would love to hear her, respond to her instinctively with the same spontaneity with which she laughingly calls to me, to show me things, to share. That magical time of children developing is such a delight – my favourite time with my own children was the 18 month to about 3 years period, when they're so curious, so interesting, so unpredictable and so very impish. My granddaughter, so unconditional in her acceptance of me, will go through all this and I won't hear a thing. Of all my losses, this grieves me the most.

#

And so to that sound of silence: my very own Tale of Tinnitus. As it becomes apparent that my hearing ability is in decline, I have thoughts of unimaginable silence, a still loneliness of my own and the disquiet of not being able to hear the baby cry. With tears and trepidation I anticipate the replacement of tranquil, natural sounds of the rain and of bird song, all the sounds we take for granted are likely to be swapped for a heavy, leaden silence.

But that silence never happens. It doesn't occur to me that the tinnitus, which crept up just as the thief did originally, is responsible for my not hearing. From being told at initial testing that my hearing was moderate, it has now dropped 20 decibels and the tinnitus has increased. The noise is unbearable. It is like a constant rushing sea or gale force wind that just never stops. I remember childhood stories of howling winds and moaning gales, exhausting to battle through ... and this is what is now played out in my ears. Each day is spent in a battle to overcome the storm, to hear and respond to the snippets and snatches that careful lip-reading helps me to make sense of and then respond sensibly to, with the words I have, rather than the words I want to use but can't remember, none of which I can hear myself saying.

What's more, there is no break from it. It's like one of those noises, a sander or coffee machine that you forget is constant until it is turned off. Except this can't be turned off. There is no silence; it feels like the noise within both ears meets at some spot in the middle of my brain to create further headaches. No music, no TV, no radio, no chatting on the phone, the only birds I hear are the irrepressible, innumerable local seagulls. It seems they have a certain pitch which, literally, just goes through me. It's a sound I can hear and also feel, physically. I should be grateful for it I suppose, but within the screech of a local Herring Gull there's some kind of eerie echo of a thief's taunting laughter.

The noise in my ears is not just tedious, it's embarrassing. I can't get my head around the fact that it's in my own ears, surely everyone must be able to hear it? It's not just whispering to me, it is railing at me. I get so confused sometimes by what's the tinnitus and what's real, thinking that everyone can hear what I hear. More than once I've asked "can you hear that?" but the answer's always "of course not!"

There's a curious cause and effect at play too, a little tinnitus tease, if you will. I always know if my anxiety levels are increasing, long before the usual bodily signs, because my tinnitus starts to rage and roar, which of course makes it even harder to hear and so inevitably makes me even more anxious about missing out on vital information, and so it goes on. And on. And on ...

#

I'm starting to really dislike my hearing aids. Each morning, after my shower, there's a whole routine of putting all my appliances in place, like a proverbial pack horse with all the bits strapped on. I put in the hearing aids, snuggle on the loop attachments then I set the right ear to two bleeps and do the same to the left.

Today, when I try do the left, there's no sound. I decide that the battery must have died, so I go to change it, then try to sit and get comfortable for a bit, but still it doesn't work. I must have got muddled, I must have misplaced a dead battery amongst the odd ones in my box, so I open a new pack instead. Two packs of batteries later I have to admit that it is not the hearing aid, it is my ear. My last bit of hearing seems to have deserted me. This realisation is almost a physical shock, which strikes somewhere mid-breath, creating a shiver across my shoulders and a tight band around my chest. Oh the shock of realizing that as bad as the hearing aids were at least there was some choice. Now that choice is gone and I'm still waiting to go to Tooting.

I can't do anything about it, but I won't just do nothing about it: I can't just accept it, so as soon as possible, the very next day I go to the hospital and manage to get an appointment with my regular ENT doctor for the same week. After an anxious wait, this latest hearing test shows that my hearing is no worse – the problem with the hearing aid must be my fault. Funny how someone pointing out your own ineptitude can feel like such a relief but given the choice I'd rather seem stupid than lose any more of my precious hearing, so at this point, I'm nothing but relieved!

The doctor is kind about it so I ask again about the medication that was suggested on my last visit. I declined it then, as the side effects are headaches and it's not like I don't have enough of them already, besides which I'm trying to get away from paracetamol and additional tablets. However, despite trying acupuncture and herbs instead, the noise in my ears still rages on and leaves me in tears sometimes. He kindly gives me the prescription. He says someone will be in touch to follow up about the hearing aids.

When I get home, the first thing I do is e-mail my herbalist to check the medication is compatible with what I'm taking from her. The one thing worse than contra-indications of meds is contra, contra-indications ... I'm having enough trouble as it is!

#

Just before Christmas 2008, my first Christmas back home, as the new me, without the sound of sleigh bells, carolling and laughter, I lose a hearing aid. I'm convinced that it's here, somewhere in the house. The first one fell out of my ear while I was on the phone but I didn't really notice, which I suppose is a reflection of just how little they do help me. It's not until I take the other one out at bedtime that I realise the first one is gone. I remove the one I have and put it on the bedside table, ready for the morning.

#

When morning comes I remember seeing the aid on the bedside so I go off in search of the missing one, which I find on the floor, beside the phone. I put it in its box so I know it's safe, but when I go to put the other one with it, I can't find it, even though I know I put it on the bedside. Once again all my positivity and effort towards the time of year is weighed down by my own anxiety which overtakes everything. I'm on full, obsessive alert looking for it and the more anxious I become, the louder my ears roar their dis-concerto! Sam comes over to help me and despite the two of us carefully searching, there's no sign of it. But I know it's here, deep down I know it's here somewhere.

Not that me knowing anything for sure counts for much, because I never can be truly sure of anything anymore, so the rigmarole starts with a trip up to the hospital to make an appointment to get it replaced. Unfortunately, to do so I have to work with the lady on the desk, who proves to be the least helpful person I've met so far in my dealings with the hospital.

She tells me that a replacement will need to be paid for and that another one won't be issued until I pay cash or cheque.

"It's OK," I say, "I just want an appointment."

She gives me 6th January, which she says is the first appointment available, what with the Christmas break and all. So, while I wait I will have to manage with just the one. Sure, I know I'm not a hearing aid fan, partly because I've found their effectiveness to be so limited, but I don't like the idea of not having them. Once again, it feels like someone is just snatching away at the few choices I have left.

I try to get on with day-to-day things in the meantime, including getting myself a bit groomed and presentable for Christmas celebrations. Over a week later I go to the bedside drawer to get my manicure set out and to my surprise, lo and behold there, caught in the closing of the pouch, is my hearing aid. The relief is enormous and all encompassing. It's hard to explain to anybody what I go through when something like this happens to me – the emotional effect equals any national disaster because I can't rationalise it at all: I shake and fret, the tears flow and I feel so frustrated. People try to be helpful and say "it will turn up" or "you can get another one." To me that is little help and even less comfort as the search in my head / mind is constant, and waiting to get appointments to organise replacements only adds to the frustration. But I've come out on top this time in two ways – I was right in my conviction that the aid was there all along and at least now I have two aids for Christmas.

#

This referral to St. George's is the start of a whole new aspect of my life, another aspect of the whole new me which, in truth, has become very much a quest for damage limitation.

This first morning, I see a hearing therapist, who's very nice and very thorough. I end up with her for over an hour, part of which is spent with her filling in a pre-appointment questionnaire that I should have received in the post. She talks a lot about coping strategies and skills and asks with genuine interest about this low level noise, my tinnitus.

Then she says that there the White Noise Generators, which are worn like hearing aids but produce an alternative sound to counteract the noise of the tinnitus. She tries to demonstrate this, using a model to show what she's talking about. She says (and shows me) that she thinks whatever is going on is past the inner ear and she will refer me to an audiology physician who will further investigate what's happening in my ears, so that the most appropriate treatment can be decided upon. It all sounds reasonably pro-active and positive and I feel heartened, understood and a little less isolated.

However, this feeling soon slips away as she cautions me not to expect any significant changes even with treatment. Like a soothsayer, she warns me of the long road ahead, in the context particularly of what my body has so recently been through, the very complete shock to my system of the Viral Encephalitis.

"Do not underestimate what has happened to you" she advises. I confess that half the time I'm still not really sure what has happened other than it has robbed me of life as I knew it, that my clock has just stopped.

In the meantime, she fits the white noise generators, although they are more sitting, than fitting, in my ears. She suggests that I go back to my local audiologist and have open mould ear pieces made for a more sure fit.

So, I leave her with a trip to my local audiologist pending and an appointment with her audiology physician on its way. Today's appointment is not the end of the road just the beginning of another chapter. Although Sam has kindly brought me here today, with a small baby and some post natal issues, this is clearly neither practical nor good for her.

Nor for me. However, with a strange sense of symmetry, as my hearing issues develop with alarming speed and the appointments become more frequent, so my strength and endurance start to increase, as if to compensate for the need for these trips.

#

So, as time passes, I venture to St. George's by myself, by train. Regaining the ability to do so would be exhilarating, if the whole thing wasn't so exhausting and so frightening. Every time I'm on the platform, with the noise in my ears rushing through my head, I seem to catch a glimpse of the ghost of myself on a platform past, with a noise raging in my head as the thief climbed aboard at the very start of this journey. This happens every time and terrifies me anew.

#

It's January 2009, almost a year after being first struck with VE and I am attending my appointment for the open moulds to be created. I've had the white noise generators in my possession since the very end of December 2008 and have hardly worn them as the fact they don't fit properly makes me far too paranoid and anxious about losing them to (a) try to wear them (b) receive any benefit from them if I do try to wear them.

At the appointment, I'm asked when I lost my hearing aid, so I explain that was found and this appointment was made later, for moulds. This apparently is not what's on the notes, so the practitioner has to go to speak with the Head of Dept.

When she returns she is content that the issue is resolved. "It's OK, it's a 216 we need!" apparently, but a 216 turns out to be a process which will now take 3-4 weeks! She fills my ears with a plug on a thread then pumps in a syringe full of something that sets and takes a mould. I come away tired and tearful. I feel my hearing has got much worse since the weekend, just from trying to do too much, just from trying to stay on this very long road.

#

I'm called back in February to finally get the open moulds fitted so that I can use the white noise generators.

This time, I see a different ENT doctor, who's friendly enough but perfunctory. My hearing test shows no change, I now have the open moulds, so what more could I possibly need? I don't need to be seen again for a year ... one Dept finished with.

#

In the fullness of time spent in a sensory void I am registered deaf ... a card in my purse to acknowledge a hidden disability, to join the one from the Encephalitis Society on ABI. They don't do cards for incontinence and memory loss, otherwise I might have been able to get a full set.

However, what this registration does grant me is, literally, access to grants. After almost two years of deafness and long after I am forced to sell my business due to my regretfully declined state, I am granted a grant from the Access to Work service for a radio aid and an adapted telephone. For me this is a big breakthrough, but one I feel I deserve. I can't help but feel the grim irony of the grant name though.

#

One thing, which has come alongside many aspects of my impaired self, is that the quest for solutions and repair leaves you vulnerable to so much opportunistic marketing. I've been a very savvy business woman in my time, but this new me finds herself suckered into applying for an amplifier for the TV, which I find advertised in sympathetic and soothing script in the newspaper. It's clearly a con to get you in for an exclusively resourced hearing test but of course I don't realise this until I am in the chair. My "before" situation is tested and then I receive a demonstration, a glimpse of what my "after" may be if I can bring myself to part with a cool £2,500 – for each aid!

This "after" really affects me. I don't pretend to know what the technology involved is or, importantly, why it hasn't been even alluded to by those NHS services I've visited, but I become very emotional when it's demonstrated to me by this company that actually, after all this time, I *can* receive an amplified level of hearing which doesn't also amplify the tinnitus! This is as close to the sound of my old self that my hearing has offered for a long while, but it comes at such a huge cost, one I can't afford.

I'm going to think about it though, I tell them, but away from this high-tech sales pitch. However, my first stop isn't the bank, it's going to be back at the audiology clinic to check if the aids I have can be adjusted any further. Which of course they can't, the limitations of the NHS provision are spelled out to me, just as the tantalising echo of hope slides out of price range.

#

Of course, becoming hearing impaired doesn't mean you lose the sense of wanting to listen, I guess in the same way that amputees complain of wanting to scratch an absent leg. I still get those days when, in my previous life I could have put on a CD and sung my heart out while driving or doing battle with the vacuum cleaner. Now I can't remember what I used to sing or what songs sounded like or, come to that, what I sound like.

Sometimes I will myself to make it happen. I turn on the radio and take a tough stance with myself: if you try hard enough you will hear it. Like a child in wonder at a new invention, I sit with my ear close to the radio, with excited anticipation, until my resolution is knocked asunder by something tougher, uglier: the storm in my ears. Then, and only then, do I accept defeat and turn the radio back off.

#

Then there's the lost art of conversation. This in fact summarises one of the worst aspects of being deaf. Forget not knowing that someone's banging on the front door to be let in whilst I'm oblivious to their presence, because once they're in the house, what kind of conversations do we have anyway?

The fact is, being deaf impedes your conversational skills, you're no longer involved in conversation in a way that matters. This takes several forms:

* When there are more than two of you, then it doesn't matter to the other two – they can talk to each other.

* Sometimes, more often than you'd like to think, people just don't bother. But I've learned that a

companionable silence only works if one of you is happy to be there, without the sound a joy of conversation. If you're sitting there with tinnitus tones raging, hearing aids whistling, unable to remember anything exciting to talk about, then silence isn't golden, it's tarnished tat.

* You're only told or included in what's necessary, such as plans and instructions.

* Non-verbal communication is decided on as an option. Instead of looking at you so that you at least have a chance to lip-read, others look away and point away, into the distance, or is it to something close up? Who knows? Without the lip-cues I can't be involved in non-verbal communications either.

#

My sister says to me that I seem down, quite a lot of the time. I ponder this. I think, yes I am, but then I know I'm not, not really down, just detached and isolated from any sound or occurrence other than tinnitus. Closer to the truth is the fact that I'm bored: being deaf is boring. I get bored by myself trying to make conversations commenting on the blossoms, the daffodils, the flower beds – there is no subject in my head other than what I see, apart from little snippets of recollection which interrupt my visual memory and add to the confusion.

#

Even though I have an adapted phone it is sometimes impossible to work out what people say when they are on the phone and particularly if they call from a mobile. When I say "I can't work out what you are saying" the standard response is: "oh it's a bad signal!" Er no, it's a deaf person at this end actually.

Sometimes, I can hear their volume but the diction is poor and then people shout to try and compensate. So I just hear more volume and even less diction. It's frustrating to the core, but it's also frustrating to say and then have to keep saying, "it is not the signal, it's my ears. I just can't frigging hear." Or in the bank when the teller insists on looking at the desk or computer so I have to say "I didn't hear you, I'm deaf and I need to lip-read" to get them to look up.

They do this affably, usually with a cheery "that's OK" and I want to shout "it's not frigging OK, it's a huge loss to me!"

At other times, I can hear volume and nuance, but the speed people speak at makes it impossible to hear and process in a single moment. Mostly, people speak very fast and leave me blinking in wonderment as I try, hard as I can, to take it in.

So this is the sound of my silence, the effect of my thief, the roar in my head. People think that I am managing, but what they think is managing is actually maintaining a constant struggle. Deafness is not a passive impairment, the thief has taught me this.

23. Coping, Caring and Feeling Crap

Once I'm home again I am deemed to be, by and large, significantly recovered. On the face of it, I suppose I am because things are 'in hand' medically, but the truth is, I'm not so much feeling well as feeling disturbed, really. My list-writing is still as obsessive (and vital) as usual, but I'm finding myself now also writing a lot of poetry.

I sit with any old scrap of paper, any nearby pen or pencil and it pours from me, as if from nowhere but clearly from somewhere. I'm spending a lot of time on one particular poem 'The Woman I Used to Be' and I'm sure it is she who is writing the poem.

Of course, 'writing' and 'poetry' are both words of overstatement when it comes to my scribbled outpourings. They're better described as scrawled, unintelligible notes which I try to convert into a verse. This rarely works because half the time I can't find the words I need: I readily tap into my emotions but the expression, the lexical definition of them eludes me. I'm barely able to cobble together something which reflects my feelings, but I'm adamant that it should make sense to me, that these expressions should somehow have rhyme, rhythm and flow: all those aspects of my life which are, in fact, still largely missing. I get distracted too, from my labours (the incontinence has a way of doing that) so I break off, wander off, sometimes paper in hand, sometimes abandoning it on my way to whatever chore, whichever place. When I return I then become preoccupied with finding the paper, it's as if someone else has removed it.

I now live in a house of secrets and lies
Cryptic messages on the calendar appears
Yet others may know but I must not hear
Unable to distinguish between what's fake and real
Invitations have ceased from family and friends
And who has been in my room?

#

Just as, over time, I noticed that aggravations and intolerances improve when I maintain a certain distance from family, I'm now noticing a direct link between my writing and those times when family distance is of the very close up, intensely personal kind. When things are said which, to me, are extreme or not what I want to hear, I retreat, tissues in one hand, pen in the other to write and cry, cry and write.

Dear child of mine
I have to move on as it's very clear we don't get along
I do appreciate all that you have done
Tho' you think I don't see you and all you have done
Who can't see who - you know I am right here
And my love will always be here
Who cannot see who?
You or me?
Maybe it's you that is missing seeing me
And do what you think not what you feel
How I hate this disease and what it has done to me
Bereft of the person I once had become
I miss my mouth and drop my food
This seems so very rude
Now just a shadow of who I used to be
And I wait for what's promised and never dare hope
My gait diminished, my speech eroded

Everything that bothers me becomes a poem or an attempt at a poem. In the absence of someone to talk with, or after the presence of someone to talk with but who holds no ability to listen and to understand, I write. I write even if these scribbles do not make any sense and are barely legible. I write to cope. Yet, despite all my work to try and make sense, on paper, of what's happened to me, what's still happening around me and to me, I still fall short of being able to explain it, explain myself.

No matter how many times people tell me how well I am doing, how strong I'm getting or how much I have achieved, it only goes a small way towards my own acknowledgement of myself – I still don't want to be here or have to do this. I'm still very much not the woman I used to be, the woman I want back.

#

I might not be too good at poetry, but I'm getting better at coping. I try so hard to forget my limitations that, at times, a measure of success creeps in and I find myself plodding along pretty darn well, actually. But, like a shooting star, the moment flashes by and the physical strength, energy or alertness is suddenly burned out and I find I don't have the physical momentum or ability to carry on, finish up what I started or even to tackle a particular task. Alternatively, I might set about some jobs and sit down to do them. Sometimes, when sitting, I forget my imperfect body, which is good, but when I get up to move I'm suddenly reminded by my imbalance and dizziness, or the screaming stiffness of my muscles. This shocks me back into the Encephalitis stage and makes me realise what a fragile thing recovery is and how disability, even disguised as a "relative" wellness, can be so pernicious.

#

Coping has a bed-mate of course ... acceptance and there are times when I struggle with one as much as the other. Some days, I even manage to accept this raging in my ears, preferring to believe it will leave me again one day and that one day I will hear my granddaughter when she speaks to me. How I would love to hear her ... I don't want to believe that I'll always have to say to her "Evie, can you look at me, Grandma can't hear you?" The poor little mite, she apparently says "sorry Grandma" so many times, or "please Grandma" clearly feeling reproached or denied, when all I am trying to do is establish what she is trying to tell me.

#

There are days when I can't think of anything - words to describe something. I know that I know them but they won't come. Sure, everyone has their tip-of-the-tongue moment, but the words I need don't get that far, they're nowhere near the tip of my tongue, even after all this time it's like back in January where the search of my brain for Evie's name turned up nothing except "baby girl." It's like I don't even know what I'm saying, what I'm talking about, where to begin the search for the words, the description I need: I feel totally uneducated and ignorant on a bad memory day.

#

I still go back to the clinical psychologist, for a significant time throughout this, my on-going 'recovery' period. I lurch from those early days of her intervention, when once a month is just not enough when trying to cope alone, even though I am so reluctant to actually go. However, at some point I realise that I do indeed need her support. She says that this realisation is progress in itself. Really? I'm not sure that the fact I realise I still feel crap about this whole business is actually a step forwards, but by her definition it seems to be.

We talk about progress a lot in the course of our sessions. She sees my search to make progress – both the intangible and the impossible kind. She's the person to whom I off-load my convictions about wanting to hear better, when I believe there is still hope of hearing. She's the person with whom I have to work through the fact that I then find myself referred to London and registered as deaf, my hope of progress now not measured by my ability to hear, but by her own measure: my reaching an acceptance of the fact that I can't. I guess we achieve a kind of compromise. In my efforts to cope with the deafness, the acceptance of it has to creep in there somewhere too. It is the process of accepting the fact, but with the vague hope that the tinnitus storm still might just blow itself out at some point, just stop.

We talk a lot about support systems – more coping with feeling crap, internally or with others, those who care about me, for me. These discussions take place across any area you care to choose, like a checklist: still deaf, still incontinent, still frequently in pain, still can't remember so yes, still needing support. There's also the other level of support needed, to cope with the bombardment of, well all of these changes, all of which need processing and dealing with in some form: the isolation of deafness; the embarrassment of not being able to hear; the fear of smelling; the randomness of getting the virus. She says, "If you moved a fraction one way or the other would you have missed it?" Would I?

So this is therapy to help me cope. And I cry. A lot. Whenever I cry I feel I'm back at the start again but deep down I know that's not so. At that time I was hardly able to walk up her stairs, but now I have a basis for comparison of my own ability to cope, to progress. Of course I still can't run up her stairs but I can manage much better, much more independently of support. Her stairs seem to be a metaphor for her intervention, including the fact that they're straight up and down, for, if nothing else, being here in therapy gives me permission to be me as I am, no pretence, no expectations.

So this is progress of sorts. But of course I'm insatiable in wanting it all to be over with, all to be 'fixed' ... this is the progress I crave in the other areas of my life. I feel that others should be able to see when I am in a dip, but they just say "you're just tired" or "you look tired". This is when I want to scream, "I feel crap! I'm fed up, I have been for weeks, but no one notices and no one talks with me, so how would you know?"

This is the question, how *would* you know? I'm physically upright, so the world sees what the world wants to see. It's not even the Emperor's new clothes anymore, the Emperor isn't even in them, it's a mannequin, still broken, just a façade of a person who, just like those clothes, is completely non-existent. So, passive mannequin that I am, I'm just told all about what others have been doing, with rarely a break to get a word in, let alone to be asked what I'm up to at the moment, or have been doing.

#

My sister comes to stay quite often, as she flies over to attend a class in East Sussex, she pops across to visit me whilst she's here. My appointments of course continue and so she has the dubious honour of being the person to drive me to a workshop being run by the clinical psychologist. There will be seven of these sessions, each two hours long, at the hospital, my least favourite place in the world. I really don't want to go, but my therapist has really been adamant that I will benefit from attending, so here I am. Regardless of what I really want, it's just like my use of other therapies ... the bottom line is that I will seek and attend anything which claims the possibility of benefiting me physically or emotionally.

However, this group is a bigger thing than I thought and I almost want to go straight back out the door. There are about 15 women and 2 men, all crammed together for this first getting-to-know-you session. Somewhere I recognise a dark thread of humour in the situation: a getting-to-know-you session for individuals with memory problems! Hmm, how many faces will be familiar next time around, I wonder?

We have to work in small groups and write down our hopes and fears for the group, share what we want to get from the group. In many ways I feel sad when people's priorities come back as wanting to help their families cope with them and their illnesses, whether it's Parkinson's, Multiple Sclerosis or strokes. All of us, a ramshackle collective of Acquired Brain Injuries, all with the idea that our families' coping mechanisms are more important than our own. Some of them seem to have so much to cope with, it pains me. Surely their families could get other support, rather than the onus being on these patients, these people so very broken themselves?

I share my personal goal which is to get back behind the driving seat and drive by 8th December. The psychologist asks me if I've booked any lessons to which I answer a slightly confused "no." One of the men tells me he'll ask me the same question next week, another person for me to be accountable to. If either of us remembers, that is.

#

Whilst I know I am making progress and am grateful for each new achievement it's mornings like this when I trip up the stairs and burst out crying which throw me. A few days of bed again, of headaches, of feeling so tired. I want to be exhausted from doing things, not exhausted before I start.

I'm also tired of waiting. Waiting to sort things out the meeting with the accountant, waiting for returned emails just to try to meet up with friends for a coffee - it all gets too much, relaying all this information by email rather than a simple phone call.

And with the bad days, come the bad dreams: a rat attacked me, in my very bed. Bizarrely it had a G-Ramp up to my bed, so it was everywhere, all over me, all over my dream, my subconscious, leaving me exhausted and scared.

#

Still, I'm coping and coping isn't too far removed from hoping either and these two go hand-in-hand across most of my days. I pray I'm doing the right things, even though I realise that my options are as limited as my abilities. How things have changed – from the me I used to be. I know I am not the same, I don't feel the same and I'm not treated the same, even though so few – virtually nobody, in fact – has said I am different. Ah so, I know though, by the way they react to things I say and do that they see the difference too. I just have to hope I'm getting away with it, with not being me.

I also still harbour the thought that I'll wake up one day and it'll all be over: the tinnitus would be gone; the incontinence will have blessedly corrected itself; the body pains will have lifted – no body pains, no headaches, no stiff neck, no bloatedness, no turkey cock red neck. See, I can hope, can't I? I can't be accused of not thinking positive ... and you know by now how I feel about being told to do that!

But I guess I know it won't really happen like that, in truth it's just not happening like that. It is all so slow, I have to remember January, February and March – those evil worst months and use these to recognise physically how far I have come since then. Yes, OK, it's good ... but it's not good enough for me. I want to be better, fitter. I want to be able to do a day's work and not need to be in bed at 8pm, plus having to pace myself the next day. On that next day I want to get up in the morning and do the same all over again, just like the woman I used to be would have.

#

The second psychology group takes place. I have mixed feelings about it, both before I go and during the session. We have to do a life graph, in as much as we can remember our milestone moments. My feedback, when asked, was that in the main although my downs were bad, in general I had more ups. Although my memory's not to be relied upon of course, I'm fairly sure I have the main parts right.

For some reason, I become very emotional as I talk through my time-line, this is me and the woman I used to be, all mapped out together. I'm almost inconsolable as I talk about losing my baby nearly 40 years ago, but the others are supportive. It's a nice group, a fair mix: some people talk a lot and others not much. I miss hearing a lot of what is said but I get by.

Just as last time, I'm struck by the number of us, a group of individuals with a serious amount of physical and emotional 'baggage' to deal with between us, who are more concerned about our relatives and how *they* are coping, than about our own recovery. The two issues are so closely linked it's scary and is again food for thought as to why it's so important that families are supported to know more about devastating conditions such as Encephalitis. Even grown up children, such as my own, could be supported to better manage their fears and the unknowns which come with the condition.

#

Preparations for Christmas are on the cards. People are talking about their events, their Christmas "do", their holidays, their plans. To anyone else it might seem selfish that I don't want to share in their excitement, which I don't want to hear all about it. It would be easy to assume that my lack of interest is borne of spite or self-pity because I am so far from being able to do anything like that myself, but it's not, not at all. I'm happy for them but my lack of interest is a coping mechanism, it's self-preservation against comparing myself to this time last year, when I was in their shoes, preparing to dance.

Today I have to send my apologies of non-attendance to our Trade Association Annual Dinner in London. I haven't missed this in years, although even as I scrawl out that I "regretfully decline" I'm aware of the double-meaning of the phrase in comparison to last year's event, when the fearful headache and the strangeness of my 'self' heralded the stealthy arrival of the thief. I push the thought to the back of my mind and try to think of the future instead. Yet I can't see it … I see that thief of the Christmas past, and of this, the Christmas present. Who's to know if it will still be around in the Christmases of the future too? Who knows if I will ever be able to do these things again? I just want to hibernate, lock myself away from the time of year, yet I still push on.

#

I suppose my reflections on coping wouldn't be complete without the question of faith and its role in coping. In truth, Mass is an event of mixed emotions for me, still. I know I may not have my physical strength and I'm a shadow of the person, of the woman I was. But I should still have my strength of character, my humility, shouldn't I?

Yet here, in the church, in the place where I should be the most humble, the most grateful, I feel the most hateful. Almost with a physical force, I hate to see these pert 70 and 80 year olds at Mass, as they nip about doing the collection, or communicate in the choir while I sit, mostly, feeling useless, bereft. Here of all places I should just be grateful for what I have got.

The only explanation I have is an oxymoron in itself: it's because I feel older, so much older than these other perky pensioners, yet at the same time, because I have known so much more ability, health and freedom, this is like being pushed back to childhood to start again: to re-grow, get stronger, develop, re-learn. Today I feel it's so unfair and I think of my old boss, who would always respond to this kind of statement with "what's fair got to do with anything?" This tempers my frustration a little although if I'm honest it still rankles: I've done my share of hard work in just getting on with life, bringing my children up, ultimately alone, alongside a quest for financial survival. Why do I have to go through it all again, without even the physical and mental fortitude of the woman that I used to be to fall back on? In this place of prayers, just like in that place of beds, trolleys, machines and medicine, my questions go unanswered.

#

I suppose the therapies are a leap or act of some kind of faith. I've now attended my second EFT session in a bid to find more, better coping strategies. The therapist suggests an option of three sessions a month, which reduces the costs considerably to about half the cost per session, so I will think about it during the week. This treatment feels very liberating and very different to anything I have done before. Despite the therapy's hands-on methodology, I can't put a metaphorical finger on how it's helping me, yet to say I feel moved or emotional whilst I'm there is an understatement: I cry and cry whilst I'm in the session, which I'm sure is a very positive thing ... where else would all that emotion go otherwise? The negative is that as well as money, it also demands yet another commitment of time, not to mention huge effort from me.

That said though, I'm sure that hydro will stop soon, as will the psychology group unless we choose to meet up informally, without the therapist, for DIY support. It's that kind of group, very supportive. Today so many of us are emotional as we're required to do another exercise and talk through our core beliefs and NATs (negative automatic thoughts). This ironically leads into talking about next time being the last session. My thoughts automatically pop over to "what then?" But I can't work out if this is a negative automatic or a prevailing positive thought, to be looking ahead at last?

#

Talking about looking ahead, after a long period of list-making, discussions and anxieties, one final aside, a major but final thing to cope with comes to fruition. Today, after a long meeting, I accepted, subject to contract and certain other conditions, the offer for my business. At the end of the meeting with my accountant and prospective purchaser, the buyer has to leave promptly, to see his own bank manager and accountant. He promises to get back to us and I know that he will. He's been very reasonable so far, even over the things which I feel have dragged out because I've struggled to get to grips with them.

When I voice this, my accountant tells me, "you're being too hard on yourself." He points out that the time this has all taken has been quite usual for the sale of a business and, by and large, it's gone well "considering your health circumstances." He takes all the accounts he needs for the VAT quarter and, along with all my future prospects and the financial security I still secretly hope to wake up and find intact one morning, heads off back to London.

I am shattered into my bones and deep down, in my soul ... I just want to sleep. I'm home by 4pm, but I still have to get some dinner and make some calls. Some would say that on this kind of day, the emotional and practical implications of selling your business is enough to make you tired, but managing tricky work days is what I did before, but back then I thought nothing of getting the dinner and then planning my evening. Now all I want is to settle with my arnica cream for my joint pains, take my various other pills and potions then make my calls before bed. I call my children to let them know about the business. They are all pleased that I've made the decision to go ahead with it.

So, today wasn't just about pushing through the usual everyday physical, emotional Encephalitic mayhem, it was also about getting past a real emotional sticking point. Those pensioners, those retired ones, I'm now just about signed up to join them, although well before the appointed age.

It's not how I imagined this moment to be, the moment of freedom from work, from which I was planning to launch myself into that Third Age, that future of family, fun and travel, the moment I would finally be leaving work behind. This reality is very different. The sensation I feel isn't a tingle of excitement and anticipation, it's a creeping dread and numbness as I realise that I wasn't quite correct when I thought the thief had taken the woman I used to be whilst I was asleep, unconscious, and infected. Today, wide awake and with full consciousness and every faculty I could rally in what was a very important meeting, I know that I waved the very last glimpse of her goodbye.

24. The Rocky Road of Role Reversal and Relationships

Since being in this situation, I seem to be thinking about my parents and parental relationships more. As I'm pretty confused a lot of the time still, I can't seem to get my head around what I'm thinking, where I fit in the scheme of things and quite what the dynamics in my familial relationships are.

I cry, still cry so much and Sam still doesn't 'do' emotions but this gets caught up in my confusion: it appears to make Sam the grown up, yet I remember tears, silences and humming were my mother's currency, all well rehearsed and taught. Sometimes I catch myself within my floods and wonder now am I crying with my mother, or for her or just expressing all the childhood tears and fears that I never shed, now that the thief has rendered me infantile within my emotions yet senile cognitively and physically; a needy child trapped in an old woman's body?

#

I remember when my granddaughter was much smaller my daughter reacted extremely to something I did, by way of attention to the child. Her reaction prompted me to ask directly if she was she jealous of the attention that I was giving her.

"Of course not" she said, in sharp tones. Yet it reminded me how it was, how I felt when my father loaded attention onto her as his first grandchild, even suggesting that he would love to be able to look after a child now that the pressure of earning for a big family was over nearly for him and times had improved. Interestingly I'm stuck with a memory of around the same time reading an interesting article in the Daily Mail titled something like 'Am I jealous of the attention my mother gives my child' or something close to that, written by a young woman of approximately my daughter's age.

So "yes" is more likely the answer, especially as I've been plunged into a different physical and head space which feels happier relating to the child of 12 – 18 months old, who is helping me to learn to walk, who demands nothing more of me than just comfort and care. I guess when the occasion arises we fulfil each other's needs and, unknowingly, it is difficult to look at a mother of nearly 40 with a husband and child and remember consciously that she is my baby. Yet that feeling never leaves my subconscious: her own child being so close, physically and developmentally, feels like her rebirth as well as my own.

#

Of course I can remember that even as a small child my daughter would trigger an argument, an emotional explosion and outpouring to get it all out in the open. Oh, and it was always my fault. The last experience of this I can remember was when she went to University. With a strange parity to my own childishness, I see her old pattern of reverting to childhood behaviour. Unfortunately, I'm not now in a position to be able to see, much less deal with the little girl within this woman of nearly 40 standing in front of me.

At times, in the course of the illness and this long road of 'recovery' emotions have been a feature and certainly would be for anyone on this same road. In the heat of the moment things get said which, to me, are extreme and certainly not what I want to hear. One evening, after being finally discharged from the hospital, Sam says to me "when you were really sick and not able to do anything it was much easier … I just picked up after you and brought you some food!"

I can understand her point but not her lack of compassion: yes I am sure it was easier, as with a baby, except a baby doesn't have the loss of a lifetime's experience to contend with or a 'before' to compare with this new, hideous 'after'. I can't help but think that this situation also reflects Sam's comparison of my before and after, her own lack of ability to cope with the loss of her mother as she knew me, whilst all the while being unable to access society's support systems or any other professional help for that matter. Each of us is grieving for our own loss of me. This upsets me greatly, and when I'm upset, as you know, I write and cry, and cry and write.

You say I can't see you but I wonder why,
I see you, I see you, but you don't seem to hear,
I hear you all the while - who can't see who?

Is it you who can't see me with all my losses and trials?
I who can't walk - or talk at times?
Sure you can't see the mum that you can recognise.
Doing for you as you now do for me - role reversal- but I'll pull through.
You are fighting with me but can't you see it's the medication.
You don't hold arguments you say,
with your friend you start to say there
yet with me you seem stuck and won't let go
-and constantly want me in tow
-or to toe your line.
I thought I was here by invitation to live among a family
from what you said, not a lodger who just needs to be fed.

#

Trapped as I am, between my body and my "self", I'm starting to identify more with an old acquaintance, one whom I've had difficulty understanding previously. He's registered disabled after a debilitating illness at the age of 21, which was treated with far more steroids than can ever be considered to be 'treatment'. This steroid overload caused him to have a stroke from which he never fully recovered.

In all the time I've known him, he just hasn't seemed to want any kind of change to his routine: whatever is suggested he has an excuse not to do it and when the unexpected occurs, he tends to make a big deal of things yet in himself he is such a lovely man. Lately I'm humble, almost to the point of shame because I now understand better, through my own experience, how difficult it is to think differently, from the way you're thinking at the time.

Now I know that some people can 'retrain', yes with all same language you'd use in the context of an errant animal, whilst others are left, literally with remnants of their former selves, physically, cognitively, emotionally, their own "like it or lump it" where you actually do neither, but just wake up each day and get on with it in the hope that something good will happen. I realise now that it's all so hard to understand and accept, both by the victim of the ABI and their relatives, their friends. These well-intentioned individuals all have their perspective, they all want to tell you what to do and how to do it, but in truth I know that it's actually what they want *for* you, which isn't necessarily the same as what you are physically, cognitively or emotionally capable of achieving.

I think I understand Robert so much better because lately I've felt at a point where I almost feel a bit bullied by people telling me "do this" or "you'll be better when you ..." across all of those scenarios that could come into play as milestones towards recovery, i.e. go back to your own house, cook for yourself, get back 'out there'. The worse one of all is, when I get upset, being told to remember to do things differently next time, when actually next time is a goldfish experience: it's like the first time again. So whilst it's lovely to have visitors and company and it gets me out to do things, sometimes really pushing myself to do things, I am happy to be on my own again when they have gone. I think about where Robert has been coming from for all these years and, finally, I understand.

#

As with all things when trying to recover from Encephalitis, you can't stop measuring yourself against what you need to do and of course the measure of progress in recovery is that you're able to do them once more. From having to re-learn to use a deodorant, to read and to write, there was a point when thinking that I'd ever get behind the wheel of my car again would be just an ask too far. When it came to informing the DVLA of my incapacity, as you now know I didn't imagine I'd ever drive again, despite experts and medical professionals saying to me "of course you will."

For such a long time, inside, I feel I'm not able to and I can trot out a whole list of very valid reasons, to do with my own safety as well as that of others: I'm too scared; I can't imagine being responsible for this tank; the car just seems so big; I don't feel that I have the physical strength to handle it. At some point, when I see the neurologist and we discuss it he says that it's just a matter of confidence. "You have lost all yours," he acknowledges. "But it will come back."

#

Once I'm recovered enough to return home and once I recover from the rigours of that, the thought of driving again starts to creep in. What with my tired limbs and painstaking gait which still needs sticks, whilst my car sits patiently at the kerbside, getting back into the driver's seat seems like the ideal solution to both my mobility difficulties and the growing sense of isolation which, like the rats, pervades my days and nights. All the time I'm so reliant on medication and the watchful eye of the neurologist, of course it's not permitted but as soon as he says that I can drive again when I want to, the seed seems to be sown.

One afternoon in October 2008, during Frances's visit, we are both at my office where she is helping me, when time comes to return home. I lock the office and go to the car, letting myself into the driver's seat with an instinct which is as motivating as it is surprising.

Frances gets into the passenger seat alongside me.

"Where do you want to drive?" she asks.

"Home" I say. And so I do. It feels a little like being in a bubble, with not being able to hear what's going on around me, but I am slow, careful and diligent and it feels fine, in fact the only thing which seems strange about it is that I'm not nearly as nervous as I thought I would be. My first drive and I can tell the support group next week that I had my lesson. Part of me feels like I should be really overjoyed about this milestone but, in truth, I have been more excited about other things like being able to write or walk, so driving is no big deal in itself, although what I might now have the freedom and the ability to do as a result of getting back behind the wheel, is.

#

On the Saturday I drive again, this time with Christina. She has come to help for a few hours at my house then we've planned to carry on in the office. I ask her if she would mind me driving and she says it's fine, she's ok with that.

It is a recovery milestone, that's for sure, but it brings with it some unexpected frustrations of its own. Telling people I've been driving a little leads to an automatic assumption on their part: "Oh, that's great, Catherine's driving again." I'm glad they're happy for me, of course, but

I'm a long way off driving per-se ... I have made a start that's all and only ever with someone else, another driver beside me. Although I do think that's an achievement, I still need to do it on my own.

#

The chance comes a little later, towards the end of 2008. At some point, absently or consciously, I'm not sure which, I pick up the car key and put it on my key ring. One Sunday morning, I'm thinking about attending Mass along with my need to go to the supermarket and the fact that I often go with Sam, when she arrives at my door to say that they are off to Tunbridge Wells for lunch, then on to Whitstable to see Simon's sister who has just had a baby. I wish them a happy trip and almost immediately an unconscious plan to make a little trip of my own springs to mind. Of course doubts creep in, but I assert myself against them: I can go out if I want without a taxi, and because Sam's out of town it does not mean I have to stay in, just as I don't want them to be stuck with ferrying me around: I just want a little of my old independence, to have freedom and not have to rely on anyone else.

So with my new found confidence I throw my shopping bags into the boot, my boot, where they should be and I get into the car. Everything functions properly, even me, and I drive to Mass without hesitation or problem. After the tea and chat that follows Mass I give Pat a lift home and then join the traffic to the supermarket. It's usually a ten minute drive but today it takes me a whole hour, but not because of me. Apparently there has been an accident further on, lots of cars are turning around to find alternative routes but I'm determined that I'm not going to turn back now. Honestly too, the thought of negotiating a U-turn at this point in my newly resumed driving career is more than a little daunting, so I stick with it. I make it there and back safely, but this accomplishment is more than that, I know I am now back in the driving seat.

#

I do have some good periods, like now that hydro is ongoing. I have some really productive sessions where I'm worked hard by the physiotherapist. Of course I'm left exhausted, but invigorated as the physiotherapist seems pleased with my progress and says I am getting stronger. I still doubt a lot of what people say to me, but I trust that she's right because as she makes each exercise more difficult I can feel the physical and consequently the psychological improvements myself.

Unfortunately, in the midst of these better spells, I can almost rely on some doctor or do-gooder to slap me down, like when I felt strong enough to phone that woman who had Encephalitis, who then dismissed me by telling me if I was not paralysed or in a coma then it was "not that serious".

Today, my hydro feel-good moment didn't even last as long as getting out of the hospital. This time it's the turn of the woman in the hospital book shop. I'm waiting in the queue there with Ann, another patient from hydro, when a man with a trolley starts to head in our direction, clearly coming through. To oblige him, I move to the left although some of the queue move to the right. Suddenly, from behind, I'm manhandled into moving to the right by the shop woman. Her fingers grasp me roughly and although she speaks to me, I can't hear what she's saying, with the usual roar of my ears, the complication of stress and fear rampaging through me as she grasps me so tightly and of course she's behind me so I can't lip-read.

It takes every shred of dignity I still have, but when the trolley has passed, I hobble over to her and tell her "don't push me, there was not need to push me." I'm shaking all the while as I repeat this to her, but it has to be said. In fact, I shake for a long while, long after I'm home and safe.

#

Another notable example comes much later, as I'm trying to get back into the 'normal' way of life, of doing things. It's voting day so I go to the polling station, which is my regular one except now it doesn't feel very familiar. I followed the arrows and the first teller speaks to me, but I can't hear her. I ask her to repeat but she can't have heard me. A woman standing to one side indicates I should stay there, whilst she shuffles books of slips. I think I'm then told to move on to this second woman, but she's speaking with her face down into the desk so I can't hear what she's saying or read her lips.

"Can you repeat that please, I did not hear you?" I ask.

She looks up so I smile and tell her I can lip read, so she hands me two slips, one yellow, the other one white as she says again, "can you take your cards?"

With that the woman on the side steps forward and beckons me to her spot. She points at the two slips in my hand shows me which is for the general and which is for the local. I look at her for what seems a long time.

"Thanks," I say, "but I reckon I would have known by the names and the fact that the two black boxes are marked yellow and white! And there are all of the signs ... I am able to read, it's just her lips weren't visible and I am deaf, not illiterate."

I get through the process, but as I get myself into the car I can't hold back the tears of hurt and frustration any longer. It's these situations and such snap judgements from strangers which drive me mad. Some days it all feels too much, as even simple things can cause upset, although I have to acknowledge they would happen with or without Encephalitis, because sometimes, that's just what life's like.

25. "A Little Respect and Kindness"

One thing which always rises up out of the steaming pot of mayhem caused by the Viral Encephalitis, the resulting Acquired Brain Injury, the "shock to the system" of being so ill, the side-effects of all the required medications, oh and the peripheral concerns of losing aspects of my hearing, continence and mobility is ... the issue of sensitivity. As a result of all absolutely bloody everything to do with this nightmare condition, I appear to be quite sensitive to many issues. In turn of course this means I'm very aware when others are less than sensitive or understanding in their behaviour or attitudes towards me.

However, the problem is that although my sensitivities could be justified, given all of the above, those who might not know me so well, as well as some who should know me much better, regard all of this as me being *over*sensitive, something which has prevailed throughout my recovery.

Like in July, during the preparations to returning home. Having Frances around at this time means that I can release the tensions caused by this alleged oversensitivity, by talking things over with her and having a darn good cry as needed. Frances is, in the main, very accepting and to her my sensitivities are understandable, they don't have to be defined as an act or fault on my part, she doesn't see me as being "overtired" or having "done too much". She sees me as needing a bit of TLC, which she frequently responds to with the quiet suggestion of an early night and a cup of camomile tea. No blame, no drama, no worries. This modus operandi, of dealing with sensitivities and sensibilities comes from my herbalist's advice as to the best way to treat someone recovering from the effects of VE: "with a little respect and kindness." Unfortunately, this advice is not universally recognised, nor available upon prescription, much less passed on by the NHS as a way for families to best support someone they love who is recovering from Viral Encephalitis. Which is extremely regrettable because it bloody well should be.

#

Frances and I are having a bit of a struggle filling out my DVLA paperwork when Sam arrives. I go to put the kettle on and Sam gets involved in the paperwork with Frances for a few minutes. Little Evie starts crying so Sam stops to attend to her and Frances comes over to talk to me. All at once I'm overwhelmed. I can't help it … one minute quietly trying to concentrate on the forms, the next the flurry of noise and people all around, it's all too much. I can barely even hear what I say to Frances, much less remember what I say to her, but as soon as the words leave my mouth Sam points out that I've been sharp in my tone with her. Frances seems slightly bemused and says something to Sam, to relay to me. Sam rounds on her to "get off your backside and speak to her directly."

Quite rightly Frances does the getting up part, but quietly states that she is going out as she has nothing to contribute to this argument. She apologises for continuing to talk about the forms when the baby was crying, saying that she accepts it wasn't such a good idea. She leaves the room but Sam seems to be caught up in an issue of her own making and begins to rant about how sick of all this form filling she is.

I have to say that there haven't been lots of previous forms to be filled in on my behalf … OK, so I might have asked her to check a few letters that I've written, but masses of forms? I just can't see where she's coming from but I can see why, quite rightly, Frances is going. She's just making her way out to the garden when Sam shouts after her:

"You can walk out … I don't have that luxury!"

I think my heart has stopped. I feel myself become so colourless, I must be transparent, invisible. I'm no longer a person, just a massive pain, in and of myself and apparently to others. Throughout my illness I've always thought of Sam's actions as being to help, because that's what she wants to do, to help. Of course she has the right to say "I can't" or "I don't want to do this" but she rarely has. On the contrary, she's so accommodating in conversation with anyone we've had to deal with – the hearing people, the doctors, social worker – you'd just think that she's happy to be supporting me. But today shows otherwise. And the worse thing is that now, with Frances caught in the cross-fire, she thinks that all the family being about and seeing her upset has left her exposed. When she calms, she says she doesn't want to be seen behaving like this. There is a logical answer to that of course, but despite my own issues, I'm trying to be sensitive to hers, so I manage to refrain.

What I don't understand though is that she has such difficulty having all of herself being seen. When I've been so very upset about how I now appear to others and what they might think of this new, impaired me, my son, her brother, has quickly pointed out:

"You wouldn't be so worried about what others think, if you realised how seldom they do."

He's right of course, but I can see that Sam can't bear that she's now exposed her own frailties, her own emotional side to my shortcomings and that Frances has not only been some kind of catalyst, she's also been a witness to it. All along, when I've been emotional or what Sam would describe as overwrought, oversensitive or over tired, she's been so dismissive, telling me that I have to deal with my emotions somewhere else, that she doesn't "do" emotional.

Yet she doesn't think of that today as she expects me to deal with her emotions, which continue to spill forth, unchecked, unwelcome and, in the literal context, uncalled for. She tells me that she resents the fact that I rely on her and then when Frances comes I don't need her. I explain that it's to give her a break, yet we both know that she doesn't extend me the same courtesy, that she still doesn't think of how I feel when her best friend is with her and she does not want to see me or anyone else.

We're so caught in some kind of trap, like that Chinese finger puzzle. Pushing, pulling against each other just ties us up tighter. We have to work together on this to be free, to reach an accord, but any response on my part is now deemed *over*sensitive or not being sensitive enough. This is not the safe, secure nurturing environment that is recommended for recuperation from Encephalitis. As I'm in turmoil, trying to work out what to do next, she scoops up the baby.

"Come on Evie, let's go home … she needs a bottle" are her final words as she whips off with hardly a backward glance to myself or her aunt.

This situation between us is blaming, abusive and desperately lacking in respect. I know I will tell her I can't do this any more, because I've reached my limit. I feel too ill, too tired to have to handle these situations, which leave me wiped out for days at a time afterwards and it's not like I can prepare myself because I neither see them coming nor hear warning nuances of tones and expression. How can I re-establish my relationship with Sam, something so important to me, how can the person I now am, become the mother that I was?

#

Trying to sell my business is another ongoing source of stress and, following one buyer pulling out, I spend a dreary session with the accountant before tottering into the supermarket on my way home. Of course it's late in the year, so it's dark when I come out. Sam texts to say she's just back from a school concert rehearsal, and do I want any help? I text back no, but tell her I'll call in on my way home. I want to update her on the sale falling through and keep her in the loop.

When I'm there and pass on the news, she says "well, you don't seem too upset about it!"

She's right of course, in the scheme of things I feel I've got bigger things on my plate. I reply that she's right, I'm not nearly so upset about it as I am about my hearing disappearing. I ask her whether she got the text I sent her on Saturday night, as she didn't comment.

"There isn't a day goes by that you don't mention your hearing," she replies, simply. I know I should let this go, but it's too hard, my hearing impairment is the source of so much isolation and physical pain, I can't believe she doesn't understand this. I try to explain to her how difficult it is and she launches into a lecture about how I should keeping my head up, engage with people … it seems she's furious with me and somehow I've opened myself up to being told all about it. I'm all at sea and can't stop crying, not least because my hearing's such an emotive issue, but also because of why I came around here to start with: the sale of the business and of course everything to do with my reasons for having to sell. On top of all that this week has also seen a pharmaceutical straw for this particular camel: another reduction in the steroids, so another period of chemical adjustment. The floodgates are open and I'm inconsolable. It occurs to me that although my herbalist prescribed "a little respect and kindness", I'm not the one who needs telling.

#

It seems I just can't get on with the practical and ignore the emotional, it doesn't work for this person I'm left as. Trying to be non-emotional in order not to be criticised is too difficult for me. I'm very aware that by asking for help, I open myself up to all of this. So I decide that I'll treat myself with a little respect and kindness: I'll ask twice for help and then if it's not forthcoming, well I'll just get on my own way or ask someone else. I won't ask again as it feels like begging, which makes me lose respect for myself, something which I'm trying very hard to regain.

#

As well as a little respect and kindness, the other thing that the NHS should take on board and pass on to those who are supporting loved ones recovering from VE (or any other ABI for that matter) is a little understanding. It's hard enough for the person themselves to understand their condition, so it's not a case of understanding them or the condition per-se on their behalf, but of showing understanding that sometimes all these symptoms, all the stories of who else has had this, done that, can be so overwhelming. Sometimes there just seems to be no understanding, no time to just listen and nod.

My incontinence situation just runs on and on, so to speak. I spend a day and night at Sam's and try three times to tell her about the latest idea for treatment of this: self-catheterisation. I really do want to discuss this – it's another of those damned if I do and damned if I don't treatments, whereby making one thing "easier" gives me another thing to do, or see to, or be aware of. I really need to talk this one through.

So I try, but each time something always interrupts the conversation. One of these things seems to be an urgent need of Sam's to share with me the situation of her colleague from school who has an Ileostomy bag fitted and how well she's doing with it. I wonder how Sam can know so much about it because she seems to find it so much easier to talk than to listen as she's happily sympathising with this woman and talking about how good humoured she is. Now I understand that this lady's in the very early stages of her treatment and I truly wish her well, but I can't help but wonder if she will still be so cheerful, poor lady, when she's had a considerable period of time having to deal with "extreme" toileting issues which are not of the norm? I hope it's cured for her long before that, that she retains her cheer, God willing. But I wonder, how deep does it run, her own humour? After all, when faced with the fearful emotional flipside, humour is a mask we can all wear, when the joke's on us or tears are just too darned inappropriate.

Sam's insensitivity always shocks me, I can't help but find it unbelievable at times. However, things are ok between us just now so I just let it ride. But maybe it's not to do with relationships, it's to do with the topic of conversation? I find that no sooner do I tell my sister about this next, thrilling chapter of the incontinence story, than she's telling me about a woman who had the same complaint with her bladder causing her kidney infections! I then realise again that Sam possibly just doesn't want to know: she is unable to cope with this idea of her mother being in a similar position. I have to show understanding and bite my tongue, the sensitivity needed is all mine to show.

#

Before long though, Sam drops by on her own for an evening. This is lovely because it seems like the first time she has come to see me on her own since Evie has been born. Of course I might be wrong about that, because of my memory, what with everything happening just after Evie was born, but I honestly can't remember the last time she was here without husband or child. I just never see her alone, so it's a delight, a real treat.

We chat for a few minutes and I tell her I was just making out my list of questions for my GP after my tea. We have a cuppa and once again the unfinished story of my London appointment comes up so I tell her, finally, that I am in all likelihood going to have to self-catheterise as the only way to "manage" the incontinence.

"You don't know yet," she says. "You don't know what you will have to do."

I feel that she doesn't understand what it means. I reply that it would have been nice if she could just have said "sorry to hear that you have more tests and stuff to go through" or something like that.

"I'm just not that kind of person." She says. I kind of want to question this, because I know from her conversations about her colleague and on some of our occasions throughout my whole illness, that she *can* be very caring, very much that kind of person.

I tell her I find it difficult listening to her talk about the colleague with the Ileostomy - when I could have to do something similar, but I am corrected and told that her colleague's situation is different as it's due to a severe type of cancer and that her toileting issue may be permanent.

"If I have to go down that road it may be permanent for me too," I tell her. We're coming from different places, myself and her poor colleague, but the end result of medical toileting for the rest of our days seems to be our common factor.

"Well you don't know! I'm sorry I can't be the type of person you would like me to be," is what I hear next.

"Let's not go there," I say. I have to normalise this strange, unsettling exchange. "How about another cup of tea?" seems to be all I can offer.

And there it is. We cannot talk about these things which are so important to me, to our future, my future because of this wall of misunderstanding between us. I truly thought that Sam and I had got over the differences we had when I was first sick, but at times like this I feel there is a gulf that has not healed. I know that some of this is on my side, that I am stuck in my own world where I'm oblivious to nuances which, as her mother, I might otherwise be more aware of and definitely more sensitive to, such as the baby blues, for example. This impasse is something else the thief has taken, or left behind, I don't know which. All I know is that between this and not being able to hear the dulcet tones of my granddaughter, I don't know which of these I grieve over the most and which of us, Sam and I, is grieving the most for the loss of the mother I used to be.

26. Handbags, Gladrags and Catheterbags

This seems to be the right point at which to explore that other, excruciating but 'hidden' difference between the woman I used to be and the woman I am now: the incontinence. At some stage, between those early spells of wakefulness in the hospital and wandering off to visit the toilet in response to my clenching, moaning insides and my later, high-dosage wakefulness on other wards, I lost my continence. I don't know which ward I was in when the thief stole it, but it went all the same.

It starts off as still having that urgent need to 'go' but with no ability to do anything about it, to hold on or forestall the inevitable, which I now know to be called 'urinary urgency'. In the scheme of things, my physicians don't pay too much attention to this, apart from a supply of pads in the hospital and the recommendation to buy some Tena pads until things "settle down." Ahh yes, "settle down" - if only I'd known that this phrase held the same timeline of truth as that "fortnight's recovery"!

#

My early days at Sam's are focused around meal times and toileting issues as I've mentioned before, just like the baby. Our respective behinds are raw and sore with something we can't control, our odours inexcusable in polite society but acceptable in her case. In my case, I absolutely can't bear the thought of smelling, which is why the exhausting quests with showering and 'dealing with' the issue stay such a feature of my days. Even as I progress from laying in my own filth to being up and stumbling about, the effect of gravity doesn't help so the issue of toileting takes up a large part of every day, in direct proportion to the confidence it takes away.

#

Throughout 2008 and 2009 the incontinence is a regular feature of my lists for visits to both GP and the neurologist. My GP tends to be more concerned with the frequent infections and sees that being both a cause and effect of my urinary incontinence. Certainly it adds urgency to my need to 'go' but of course this does not explain the days of the excruciating double incontinence, where I have no warning or control over any of my eliminations. For attention to this detail, the GP reminds me to raise it with the neurologist who, in turn, listens attentively. He says he will refer me to a consultant if the incontinence continues, so I have to wait, because I can't wait, if you see what I mean!

So the issue stays on my list of questions for him each time around and of course I am emotional about it each time I start to tell him about it. He looks uncomfortable if I become emotional and cry so I try not to. I tell him I'm seeing the clinical psychologist still, he says "good, good."

I share my continued distress about the pads, the discomfort, the fear and lack of confidence, everything that detracts from my overall physical progress through fear of a movement too far, an unpredictable follow-through of cause and effect. Much as I might try to be doing more, gently exercising, trying to improve one aspect of my physicality, one set of symptoms, always comes with a noxious side-effect at the cost of another. My confidence in my body remains at rock bottom, or is that soggy bottom? After one particular outpouring of distress, early in 2010, he agrees to refer me to the National Hospital for Neurology and Neurosurgery in London, as they have a specialist incontinence clinic ... yet another department to get to know. Being in this medical cycle is so new to me, a far cry from not having been to my doctor for ten years at one point a few years ago. And now? Now I am a patient across many of the departments across several hospitals, but again I'm happy to go, this could be just the help I need to get this sorted.

#

And all the while, despite my growing experience and gradually improving dexterity when 'dealing with The Issue' and using my pads and clean-up routines, at the back of my mind is the absolute certainty that I smell like an unkempt, unclean nursing home. I am up and down at least twice in the night to deal with the urgency of a toilet visit, hopefully on time but often not, so always, always wearing pads.

#

Paperwork for the appointment arrives through the post. This is surprises and pleases me, although at the same it's confusing. It seems I have to measure the ebb and flow of what's going on down below, prior to the visit itself.

When the day arrives, involving another scary, exhausting trip to London by train, I make my way to the clinic, armed with my flow charts, in and out. I spend over 90 minutes with an extremely pleasant and thorough nurse, who fills in forms, analyses and explains ... except she does keep holding a list of dos and don'ts right up in front of her face, so I'm unable to lip-read what she's saying. I just have to hope that she will actually pass on a printed copy of her lists.

Finally I see the specialist professor, the incontinence consultant. She is a lovely woman, not austere or cold, borne I suspect of the fact that she needs to encourage intimate information about bodily functions, my bodily functions, so in the manner of a lavatory, I need to be engaged!

As she checks the notes, she's incredulous about the time frame in which I've been putting up with the incontinence ... it's taken 2 ½ years to get to see her? Why, she wants to know, has it taken so long? Was it low on the list of priorities? I tell her no, it's just that the list of problems has been so very long.

Her next big question then is what is the problem with my hearing? Is it from nerve damage or brain damage? If it's brain damage this could be the cause of my plasticity as well as the incontinence. She wants to try me on a medication to help, but a side-effect is memory loss, which would be less than ideal for me, for obvious reasons! She suggests I have an alternative medication, which my GP will have to prescribe.

Before I leave, she also suggests other methods, rather than more prescriptions as a remedy for me. Not just to help with my physical management of my symptoms, including the rigours of the clean-up campaign after accidents, but also the psychological impact and the lack of confidence. Catheterisation is possible, so that I can pre-empt (or should that be pre-empty) a problem bladder and take control rather than suffer the indignities of continued incontinence. She suggests this as an option, should the medication not work out successfully. At the end of the appointment she asks me for a sample and completes another urine test. Of course, like most of my tests recently this one too suggests that I might have an infection - which if corrected could make a big difference, so her suggestion is to bounce me back to my GP and ask him to do another lab test to find out which infection I harbour. So that's it for a moment, no magic wand but more than the usual wave of a swab! I make my way to the station, for a stop-over with friends to break up my long day and journey. Even I can see the humour as I make my way to the station for the connection I now need ... Waterloo.

#

It takes another couple of weeks to get a call back from the incontinence nurse, to let me know that the tests were ok. As far as she's concerned, that's it. I wait but I have no further contact from her and no action elsewhere, having waited for this promised call. So all that charting of fluid flow and trailing my weary body for the appointments and I'm no better off, I just have to wait for the six month follow-up appointment to come around.

I happen to comment on this to my practice nurse a couple of weeks later, when I'm attending that other much loved female appointment, my routine smear test. She tells me that my doctors are retiring and that I should come to see the new doctor, to talk about the medication. It worries me that no-one has said this before, or have they said it but didn't think to check that I could hear? Either way, I see the new GP, and am given the new prescription.

#

Of course the situation lingers. Along with my good and bad body days and excruciating head days are my good and bad continence days. There's obviously a cycle of cause-and-effect at play and the more stressed I am, the worse the incontinence. When I return to the National when my six month appointment is due, I share my continued distress that the medicine has failed to fulfil any kind of magic whilst its side effects confuse any sense of progress I thought I was making. At this point the kindly consultant broaches the subject of Intermittent Self-Catheterization (ISC). I'm so fed up with the medication and its effects that

I'll try anything as an alternative, so it looks like self-catheterisation is the way to go, as it were. The consultant tells me she will arrange for nurse follow-up, in the privacy of my own home, to teach me the process and organise the provision of items.

#

In time, the dedicated professional who will follow-up with me arrives at my home. She is late for the appointment but is neither apologetic nor aware of me as a person. She is clearly here about the mechanics of the task in hand. She uses the expression "to void" a lot and I feel myself, flustered by her lateness and abraded by her manner, becoming angry and emotional especially as, like the tinkers who used to call at the family farm to sell their wares, she tips her bag of tubing and tricks onto my dining table, of all places. She starts talking through things, without once acknowledging my difficulties with hearing, let alone the processing of such vital instructions. I have to ask her several times to repeat things which she does, although she seems to be only just avoiding rolling her eyes as she does so.

Once she is gone, I regard my new toileting regime before avoiding it for the time being, by reaching for my pen and tissues and letting my feelings about her whole visit vent forth:

ISC (Intermittent Self Catheterisation)
or
The only thing she had for sale
Was how to empty my bladder without a pail?

In she bounced, for our appointment late
Talked through her hair that covered her face
My dining room table her chosen place
To display her multitude of wears
For me the table was not in good taste
Long ones, short ones, hard ones, soft ones, scented or plain
Packaging anything but plain!
Not a dress from a boutique I gain
Or a pearl on a lovely chain
The only sale she could really claim

Was to tell me how to piss through a tube into catheter, a bag.

#

And whilst these appointments go on, few of those around me remember to ask how it's going or offer an ear for me to ponder my options and progress. I muddle along with a few month of self-catheterization, trying to take it in my stride which, incidentally, has improved a little since I've been able to reduce to pad-wearing for emergency leaks rather than constant fear.

#

My lovely neighbour, Myra, asks me in for a coffee around this time and we're chatting, quite amicably and suddenly I find my eyes were leaking, just pouring silently, steadily down my face. Gently, she suggests that I've not really been myself since I started ISC. She shares that she's experienced similar problems herself and still suffers with them, so she understands what it is like, which kind of makes me cry more but from comfort, from validation, I don't feel so stupid, or so alone. Later, when I think about it, especially the whole context of the conversation, I'm reminded of a saying of my father's when tears fell. He'd say "your bladder is very near your eyes" which I guess in a way mine has been for some time now, some time indeed.

#

After these months of trial and error with the catheters I return to the National but have to see a new, different consultant and go through the history all over again. He's very nice and together we discuss my progress and various options. He expresses reservations about implants and the danger of infection with surgery and talks more about medication and what is happening for me now, how I'm managing. Of course, as if to prove my father's expression, the floodgates open and he receives my turbulent outpouring of woe, not just about the incontinence, but everything the thief has both taken and left behind.

I think it's in this moment that I realize that I have not accepted this situation at all: whilst I go through the mechanics of the catheterization and understand its benefits, psychologically I have not accepted it. The consultant is amazingly understanding about it, gently so. He tells me that people with neurological problems need more support and help to accept being catheterized, so he offers other options to assist.

Apparently, it seems, where celebrities and the well-to-do have Botox treatment on their faces, to help keep their wrinkles in order, those like me may be able to have Botox on the NHS, right where the sun doesn't shine, to help keep their sprinkles in order. To find out about this, he'll refer me to one of his specialist colleagues. Unlike many consultants though, the referral offer isn't a brush-off to get me out of the door. He can see I need more immediate help, including "a little respect and kindness" and takes me to meet the nurse I saw the last time. She's kind and understanding and tells me that the only way the urgency and accidents can be dealt with is more frequent catheterization, possibly up to 4 times a day. She tells me that it's not unusual not to be able to void naturally once you catheterize.

#

Whilst I wait for the appointment for the Botoxing to come through, I weigh up my options, desperate to talk them through with someone. It seems that even after the treatment, self-catheterization will still be necessary, plus there will still be leaks, whilst the Botox itself will have to be repeated every six months.

I really want to talk about it, woman to woman, my problems with it, my options. When I mention to someone that I hate both the catheter and the incumbent necessity to use a mirror to get used to inserting it (still not being back to my co-ordinated best, you see), she looks at me incredulously.

"Well everyone knows where their vagina is!" she remarks.

"Yes" I retort, "and everyone knows that you don't pee from your vagina!"

I decide to contact Dr. Shen, not least because I need to know if the Botox will affect, or be affected by the herbal treatments and acupuncture I still receive from her. Her reply to my email is swift, reminding me that Botox is of course a poison and that I have spent these many troubled months trying to relieve my body of a pernicious viral poison imposed upon it. Why on earth then would I choose, *choose*, to have a known poison injected into me?

This helps me to decide and I cancel the preparation for the Botox treatment, feeling slightly relieved but also, to be honest, a great sense of disappointment. Having been through all of this, becoming familiar with myself and my bodily functions in a way I'd never anticipated, I still get caught short, literally. I can go shopping and think that all is well and then suddenly have to rush back to my front door, knowing I need the loo but find that the front door's still as far as I can get. By the time I reach the bathroom it's time to strip off like a toddler, shower myself down, put my clothes in the washer, then cry. For all of these efforts there have been no magical improvements, just back to the washer and shower routine.

#

And this, is the woman I am. I keep thinking about Jean Lapotaire, the actress who wrote about her ABI following cerebral haemorrhage. When I read her book I think, here is someone who knows, who understands what it's like when something happens to your head and you feel that you'll never, ever be the same again. She would understand my poem 'The Woman I Used to Be', what it means that I'm not the me I used to be.

I've mentioned before that you could've told the woman I was by the contents of my handbag and the irony is that you can now tell the woman I've become the same way. The cards in my purse reveal my different afflictions: one from the RNID that announces 'I can't hear you'; another from the Encephalitis society saying that "I have sustained an injury to my brain as a result of Encephalitis. I might appear fine; however I may have difficulties with memory, thinking or actions. Your understanding is appreciated"; another states "Registered Hard of Hearing". This is the same purse that once held the smart business cards of an astute, capable business woman.

And now there's my pencil case. For holding all those vital implements of communication and business – pens, pencils, USB sticks, stylus for iPad or tablet perhaps?

No, in my pencil case are my catheterisation items, my nifty snap'n'use sealed packs, my wipes and disposal bags. My pencil case holds everything I need before and after, all I need do is find a clean bathroom which, when you're out and about, can be a tall order at times!

Going to the loo has taken on a whole new meaning - using the disabled facility so that I have room to, erm manoeuvre; de-robing as far as possible, coat scarf, gloves, bag there is nothing natural about this procedure, having to stick a plastic tube into my body and pee like a man. It's not easy when my balance is bad, to hover over the loo or stand on one foot, the other on the loo for easy access then hold a mirror. While you are doing all that the pee shoots all over the place until you can direct it into the loo bowl. However, without my hearing aids I cannot hear the contact of urine with water, so the first rule of catheter club is put your hearing aids in to go for a pee.

And for someone who always wore make-up, I don't think my face ever had the mirror attention that my urethra now gets! However, to move on with my life? I just have to manage it and accept it.

#

When asked what is it about the ISC that I dislike, I inhale and gush it's just everything, lack of control, the memory of years of working in the disability field: houses and homes, be they private or care homes residential or nursing, there were so few that did not smell of urine, the smell of an old woman in the church, in the waiting rooms.

Of course I hear a lot of the old platitude "oh well, it comes to us all." People constantly want to compare my incapacity with that of what happens as we age. Only I did not get that opportunity, it happened so fast.

"Ah it happens all the time, when I cough, when I laugh! Blah, Blah, Blah!" But it's not the same as I experience, no cough, little laughter for sure, no day without a pad 'just in case'. Some could (and do) say "so what, it could be worse!" But this is my problem, for me it is worse. All of my worst nightmares about being disabled centre around my recollections of those private houses, the overweight woman (in particular), the huge TV screens with miles of cable just snaking the room and that catbox tang, the sweet'n'sour, stale smell of urine. I just had an aversion to that outcome for me from the first time I met the social worker who was determined to get my TV sorted out, so I could sit there and become another smelly statistic.

Personal note: I haven't given much direct advice in this book, because that's not its purpose; this book's a reflective snapshot, mainly from the early years of my journals and journey, it's not a how-to book. However, for anyone trying to recover from Encephalitis or ABI, for whom continence is an issue, I'd really want you to learn something very early on which I didn't know about until it had cost me dearly, literally. Having taken the Tena pad recommendation as a literal necessity, I then began buying them regularly not just because I had to for the physical end of things, but because I thought the Tena brand was what I had to use, the only option open to me.

When I moved back to my home and the social worker was, very temporarily, available for advice she suggested perhaps I should ask my GP about getting pads on prescription. However, this didn't happen because my situation was deemed to be only temporary, by myself included because of course I've always been ever hopeful that I'd wake to find myself restored once more, if not in all areas then at least in this one!

However, it wasn't until much later on, almost at the point where the alternatives such as Botox and catheterisation started to come into the conversation that I found out that some local health authorities (including my own) do offer incontinence products on NHS prescriptions!

In reality, I ended up spending approximately £10 a week for over two years on Tena products when really I could have been accessing very similar items by prescription. So, if my situation is similar to yours, it's worth asking your GP surgery whether continence products are available on prescription for you, even if your own situation is also deemed 'temporary.'

27. What the Thief Left Behind

My journals and my poems continue to be a roaring, an outpouring of what the thief took from me. Conversely though, like finding yourself approaching a mirror in a shop and thinking "who's that old lady, the careworn one, who's approaching me?" before you realise it's yourself, I do find myself sometimes locked into thoughts about what it is, as much as who it is, the thief left behind.

A legacy of poor relations seems to come out at the top of the list, and it's not just my relationships with people, as a result of my clumsy communications, their lack of understanding coupled with my own lack of clarity, there are also relationships with other things too, like my relationship with sleep, for example. From the initial manifestation of the illness including the thief's rampage through my brain whilst I slept, to the steroid-induced inability to sleep alongside with my fear of sleeping in case the thief came back or the rats and ghouls carried me off, plus the interminable waking to see to my own toileting during the night, it's safe to say that my sound relationship with sleep is now lost.

My nightly patterns of sleep and wakefulness light the bedroom like a disco, light on, light off, light on, light off. Long since I've given up laying awake waiting for the ghouls to pounce, instead I busy myself, so it's not unusual to find me painting my nails at 4 a.m., it's something I can do quietly at that time.

Of course for much of my recovery period I've been prescribed sleeping tablets, which I've spent just as much time trying to wean myself off gradually. I start by making a decision to get off them, but then the night terrors, the 'what if ...' side of sleeping creep in and so I take the tablets again. At some point I decide to just let it happen when it does, so I start to just pop the tablet out on the bedside table for a few nights, ready to be taken. More and more I begin to forget to take them, falling asleep naturally instead. When this happens over a period of several nights, I decide that this means I'm OK for now, thinking positively again of course, so I tuck the pack away in the drawer. So far it seems to be working, although a natural, good night's sleep is still not a regular bedfellow for me.

#

Of course, as the Encephalitis Society literature gently points out, emotional problems can be a significant result of Encephalitis and it's true to say that the emotional deficits and exaggerations remain with me, even after such a long time. After working so hard to find the therapies which would best support my emotional recovery particularly, I'm now working through my Act III, the final scene in my recovery with the support of the Emotional Freedom Therapy. Each session always identifies something the thief has left tucked away, lurking to catch me out and the therapist is right. She'll identify that gripping pain in my side is gall bladder or blocked energy and I feel sure she is correct, I know that there is something blocked. She thinks I need to work on the word Encephalitis because just that word/name is emotive for me. So this becomes my homework: "Even though I had Encephalitis, I deeply and completely accept myself." 'Encephalitis' she says, "strips you bare - like asking you to walk naked having always worn clothes."

She's right of course but even though we're onto the thief here, the stealthy footprint remains because even if I can accept this nakedness, others can't, they don't want to see it or can't acknowledge the sight of it, so they dress me in Emperor's clothes and choose the "you're fine" view of me instead ...

I have no crutch so I am not ill
No visible sight to alert concern
Of memory poor there is no sign
A leaking bladder I try to hide
Hearing aids on both sides
A walking stick I try to resist
"You look OK, you're doing fine"
No job to say I am this ....

No questions asked

#

I see the Clinical Psychologist for quite a while, in the end. It's never without tears but it's always good to let go of some of the anger I feel towards Encephalitis. She talks about the grieving process – the ebb and flow, the feeling that you are going forward and then the full stop of going nowhere. She talks about the loss and the voids caused by the selling of my business, family moving, all residual to my own loss, this emptiness created by the thief. Where the thief left me without my beloved singing, I am now painting instead, taking art classes. The psychologist suggests that I paint out the anger. I've probably mentioned that the vacuum cleaner used to be my weapon of choice, weapon of release, but the thief left my body too weak for the vigour required, so I paint, my passive-aggressive anger.

#

Of course the thief left behind some other 'alternative' qualities too, like my list-writing, endless note-making, journals and poetry. Without these I'd never have had this access to my own journey. Although it has to be said that much of the poetry written so prolifically doesn't really make any sense to me when I reread it now, I know that at the time I had something to say, I know how important it was then, for those thoughts to be committed to paper, sometimes when it was incredibly difficult both emotionally and physically, to do so. There's always some aspect about trying to create a verse that takes the issues out of, or clarifies them, the immediate focus for me; it's a way of working things out or saying what I need to say, even when there's nobody listening. I now realise that I really should have had talk therapy right from the start, but there was so much else happening. Instead, my scrawls became the next best thing, despite the fact that much of it has a long way to go to make it readable! Now I see it as utter rubbish, these attempts at writing but I respect how the very act of it, as much as the content, has helped me to get through my Encephalitis nightmare. Of all of my poems, the one which reflects my whole journey the most, I think, is The Woman I Used to Be which was eventually finished over a period of three years.

Despite not understanding my own poems and journals scribbled in high dudgeon and low moments, when my friend Andy offers to type them up I reluctantly pass them on. Her transcriptions, along with files and folders of copious 'notes, are then passed to Katherine to knit into shape.

Despite everything else, the thief has left me with the means to tell my story.

I guess the fact that I can now write about things other than all those direct effects of the Encephalitis: the body pain; incontinence; tinnitus; walking; sight and relationships affected by every aspect of these, is all in itself part of the recovery process and of coping with what's left. Other things interest and involve me now and I become absorbed in them even though I know I will be exhausted as a result. So although the thief took so many things, I now seem to have moved to a stage where although they remain foremost in my mind, they are not dominating me or my time and effort to manage them; it seems I have either got more used to or accepting of some things and so seem better able to cope overall.

#

I don't like the darker side of myself that the thief has left me with, but I do try to manage her. I know I experience the bitter tingle of envy now, something I wasn't necessarily given to before. My sister returns from a trip to Australia. She's two years older than me, has been fit as a fiddle, always out and about, getting here and there whilst I am just here. After Australia she's planning her birthday event, then Christmas in South Africa, this is her diary, her calendar, her to-do list. the one I am left with is not so exciting: physiotherapy; check ups; incontinence clinic; ordering hearing equipment. I can't help it, I do envy her.

Oh and I still can't help it, I still maintain that sense of resentment towards those nifty septuagenarians, who spring around apparently oblivious to their aging bodies. They will get old gradually and with dignity (God willing) whereas I was aged overnight and in a way which is nothing except embarrassing and humiliating, little spared, not even dignity.

I have been left humbled and let down in turn by many of those around me, but I try not to dwell on any of it (as much as the obsessive side of the new me will allow).

Visitors came and went, first at the hospital, then at Sam's and then back in my own home. Some came frequently, others not so much and of course the nature of a visit is that it will have an end. For some, the visiting comes to an end when I appear to be 'better', that subjective better that I'm sure you're tired of hearing about by now. Those who know me best, know the truth and still visit or send cards, show they remember not just how I am, but who I am too. The thief has left me knowing who my friends are and where the positive relationships in my life are to be found.

And let's make no mistake, after Encephalitis, relationships are bloody hard, particularly the misunderstandings and misconceptions. My sister tells me that each time I do something that does not work for me, or results in negativity from others I should learn from that, try to change it next time. Yes even with dear, understanding Frances, I can't make her see that trying to remember that is impossible, because there's no thought pattern that takes me back to the last time. Each time it is a new experience, whether it's Sam flicking her head, rolling her eyes or saying thank you pointedly, to indicate that I should say thank you for whatever the transaction is ... it just does not work like that. If I have something on my mind, then that's what's there, it's all that's there and when interrupted for something else it just does not work.

Someone told me it can be similar for people who had a stroke, when they are told a significant piece of news, they can still say "pass the sugar" because that was on their mind before the other person spoke. Personally, I can understand that entirely. People seem to miss the fact that your brain has been interrupted and in my case I've lost the abilities I used to have, even though I have my Emperor's finery. Others have no concept of the mental struggle that is going on.

However, because the thief has left me with a sense, a real drive not to have unfinished ends and quarrels, up-in-the-air attitudes to commitments, I try not to allow any of these very negative effects or comments pervade the progress and positivity which is still mine, which I have earned and worked so hard for. There is that saying: life is a coin, you can spend it anyway you wish but you can just spend it once. My life, like a clock, just stopped with the Encephalitis and it has taken me over six years to get a semblance of a 'normal' life back, yes the 'So This is the New Normal?' I am left with. My coin isn't worthless, I won't let it be and I haven't done spending it yet.

#

But speaking of visitors, it's useful to note that, unlike some of my visitors, the rats and ghouls stayed with me for a considerable amount of time, about two years overall I think. That's an awful lot of fear to be left with.

#

I am still left with questions of faith both in my God and in myself. It goes through my head so much:

Now I lay me down to sleep,
I pray the lord my soul to keep,
And if I die before I wake
I pray the lord my soul to take

We always said this prayer going to bed as children and it's strange how and when things come back to mind. This prayer left me for a time but was back throughout the thief's visit and is indeed part of the legacy. Why should it resurface then? Now? Fear perhaps? Despite its presence, its message so regularly and sincerely offered, I didn't and he didn't. I wonder, after all this time, which is best?

#

With Encephalitis the clock stops, I realise this now as I recover. I've lost years of my life, in but a moment of time. I've been left catapulted into an old age which at times seems to border on senility. In the process I've been left without the career in counselling I'd trained so hard for and left jobless without my business which I'd worked tirelessly to build up. And even this process of retirement becomes a happen-stance, rather than the milestone it should have been with or without the Encephalitis.

When I finally completed on the business sale, I felt completely redundant, useless. Left without skills, hearing or money coming in, much less any other potential to make an income. I was quickly and efficiently retired, an event which passed unnoticed except for one card to mark the occasion. One card for a life-time's work. I'm still so sad that my working life finished without a proper goodbye, good luck or even a "what will you do now?" Like my disabilities, my plans and hopes are invisible to others so they don't exist: retirement became an occasion to be ignored. I caught Encephalitis as an independent business woman but Encephalitis left me a retired old lady.

28. Letting Go

This I am sure is the first time that I have felt grateful. It's the later part of a bright October afternoon and I've just been to my art class. It's 2011 and I've popped into the supermarket to fetch my usual bits and pieces and, as I leave, my own leisurely pace is slowed down by a lady moving stately as a galleon at a snail's pace. She seems oblivious to all the bodies jostling and rushing past her. Perhaps she needs to be or has learned to just ignore all about her as she concentrates on her own activity, her ambulatory movement forwards, which she does with considerable grace. She too is using a walking stick, but it's her head which catches my attention, as she has a constant and fairly intense involuntary movement as she sails along. I'm humbled as the thought springs forth that although I might have to be here complete with my list of residual incapacities and debilitating issues, few of them now visible (although that in itself is a disadvantage at times), I thank God that I do not have to cope with something like that lady. I have no idea of her condition, her diagnosis or prognosis and I do not need to know. What I do know, because it has hit me with a genuine moment of clarity and wonder, is that I am so grateful that it is not me.

#

I have listened to so many people over the last six years tell me how lucky I was/am, how very grateful I should be and all the while I think, lucky? You call this lucky? I am not lucky and will be damned if I am grateful for what, in other people's eyes, is 'getting off lightly.' Because that's it, as far as I've been concerned I've just been plain unlucky.

Now don't get me wrong ... I am grateful for numerous things but for nothing to do with how I am. I am grateful for my children, for my granddaughter, for the professionals who have treated me. For each spring day and the rebirth of life, each summer that brings a bountiful harvest and for the glories of an open fire in the depths of winter as we celebrate the most important birthday of the year, for these things I am indeed grateful.

I have great difficulty with the concept that we choose to be where we are at and that I have chosen this condition. I would not choose this for my worst enemy. It's been a feature that I've mentioned throughout my recovery period, others telling me "you could be in a wheelchair or even in a coma." I am not in either and I still do not feel any luckier for that.

#

It seems hard for people to appreciate how all this has changed my life, both in the immediate aftermath of January 2008 and across these ensuing years of constant challenge to try to be well, fulfil others' hopes and expectations, to get back to the woman I used to be.

The things all of us take for granted no longer apply, like being able to meet a friend in the evening for a coffee or a night out, it's all pretty much a thing of the past as bed at 8 or 9pm has become the norm. The entertainments of TV and music are no longer available to me. Yes, subtitles are available but with my reading still less than fluent, they take so much energy that most programmes just aren't worth it.

I do miss my reading in general and one of my favourite leisure activities of just browsing in a book shop. However, I still try to enjoy the book reviews in the newspaper, but then forget them, although not deliberately of course, it's just normal for me.

And being seen to be 'back to normal' has its own sting in the tail. Once you're beginning to manage, people don't see the difficulty with lip reading and the phone, the not being able to lift or carry, the having to ask for help or rely on it being offered, or constantly paying for people to do odd jobs - all odd jobs that I would mostly have done without thinking about. I say mostly as of course I wouldn't have been able to do some of these things pre-Encephalitis, but it's OK to say "I can't do that" when you're leading a normal life. But when your life and your self are less than normal, there just seem to be so many things you can't do that it feels like you are wanting and needing so much from everyone else, it just breeds a feeling of uselessness. The GP has often said, when you come to a point of accepting how you are it will get easier, before he goes on to say it could happen to anyone.

But this acceptance is a very big thing. What comes to mind, when I think about where I am now, is that saying "to thine own self be true." For where I am now and the journey that the Viral Encephalitis has taken me on, I can only think "to thine own self be *truthful*." For how I am now is largely the truth of my recovery. It will not get better than this, this is my Act III, which I will play out until the curtain comes down, so now seems to be all about acceptance and expectations: both mine and others', separating them and working them out before then being able to work through them. Even now, in 2015, addressing my own acceptance and expectations is my current task.

At the same time though, I'm very aware of others' lack of acceptance of some of my conditions, or even their acceptance that I continue to have health issues and incapacities at all, because of course "you look OK." However, to do this, my life is so regimented. I have to stick to a routine which incorporates many coping strategies across so many of my physical and mental issues. In the main this works well, but every now and again the effort to maintain this "OK" look is unbearable. My hearing therapist says to me "if I sat opposite you in a café or restaurant I would have no idea that there is anything wrong with you". And there's the rub. I now present myself with the not-quite grace of a swan gliding on the water, whilst underneath I'm paddling like fury, everything working hard, so very hard to keep me afloat and no-one can see how I'm struggling, a nasty legacy of Encephalitis.

#

Expectations are the other big challenge because in some ways it seems normal, fair even, to have expectations of others. I have had to learn, or should I say *re*learn, that sometimes my expectations seem "a normal too far" so I have to work on my own expectation issues and likewise respond to what it expected of me. The trouble is, six years on this can still be more than I feel able to do, at times. I continue to work hard to adapt myself emotionally, particularly (and ironically) in respect of being adaptable myself, because even after all this time, I still find it difficult when people change plans. I get so caught up with the plan itself that there is nothing else. But I am trying.

#

I have wanted to chart my progress and make sense of my journals to tell my story for so long. Getting an editor to help knit my book together has been a great decision and Katherine has been a great choice - we seemed to gel and fit together right from our first meeting. I have written this book over those long dark years as I wrote my journals, scrawled my thoughts and scribbled my indignations and inclinations whilst the effects of Encephalitis ravaged through my body and mind. The result of my musings and outpourings has been raw yarn, skeins of loose ends, knots and worn through threads, which have been knitted together to show the pattern of this illness, of these years.

In turn, I have had to edit Katherine's knitting, revisit the sore, itchy fabric of my story. This has been no easy task, transporting me as it does back to very painful, sad and lonely times of loss. There has been lots of … did I really say that? Did that really happen? In their way, the journals have been the way through, have offered up so much detail that I probably would have forgotten for good.

Of course, I could never forget that all this happened, so suddenly and that with such a swift, complete assault on my mind and body, I was changed forever. From the start I knew that I had a lot to relearn, but somehow I also knew that I would never be the same again. In the process of knitting together my book, I can now see my progress over these recent years, the results of my battle to return back to the woman I used to be. This leads to that question of acceptance: I now doubt that I will ever be that woman again and so instead I have another battle, to accept the me that is here now, even if she is completely unfamiliar to me, this woman I have created from the pieces of myself left behind.

#

And that's just the emotional side. They physical side of the story is a little easier to tell, but then not. I have more or less accepted my physical limitations and am learning to work with them and around them. What is more difficult to accept is other people's ideas about what is OK. Even after all this time, the thread of my journals reaches to the very end: that tendency for people to say that I look great and hey, I can do so much, and all the while having little or no knowledge of my difficulties in performing those day-to-day, routine tasks, the constant effort of keeping a balance, pacing myself. Others continue to tell me how I am, based on what they see, much less on what they ask because in truth few do ask, as they move on to talk about their own jobs, careers, training and yes, opportunities.

When I think about this scenario, it reminds me of a conversation a couple of years ago with a young man whose brother had been diagnosed with Multiple Sclerosis and who had rapid deteriorations. He said of his brother: "it's so hard to know what to say to him once we get past the 'you look well' and 'you seem to be managing most of your medical appointments' - that seems to be the extent of it now he's no longer able to work."

"Do you ever ask him how he is and wait for an answer?" I ask.

"Lord no!" he responded. "I couldn't bear to hear all that he has to go through."

So there we are. That is what we, as patients in recovery, as survivors, need to learn to accept, that what we are asked extends only to what is palpable for others to sit with, to manage and that this isn't a limit to how much or how little they care, more their demarcation of the limit of what they are able to cope with.

And I can understand this of course, to some extent. I've learned to change many of my own coping strategies to directly sit alongside acceptance and expectation, for myself and others, for the woman I used to be and the woman that I am now. I've learned from getting so frustrated with offers of help which did not materialise or the "we could have done that!" after the job is done.

One thing this illness, this new life has taught me has a direct reflection on what I observed in my old professional life, where I've mentioned seeing the old, the disabled, the frail just sitting and waiting. I now know why it's like this for them: it's because somehow there seems to be an attitude that if you are incapacitated you have nothing to do but wait, no matter what for, you can wait. For myself I decided after some time and much frustration that the waiting was causing me too much anxiety, so I adopted my self-preservation policy of asking twice only, asking three times just feels too much like begging.

#

Throughout everything and even now I still rely on people and I know that in this I'm very fortunate. Maggie, my lady who comes in to help me keep the house in order, my handyman (a new one as my old one seems to have retired) and my trusted Fiona who helps me with all my admin: they are all the gems in my ring not only as helpers but because now we have become good friends too, constants on the end of the phone should I need them. I'm still at it with the lists and so I keep lists of the jobs that need to be done so that when my helpers arrive they can be done. The relief of knowing it's in hand and not having to go through the frustration is unbelievable.

The medication took a lot of the blame for my frustration and impatience, yet now, without those pills, my temperament remains the same ... the long-term effects of the medications themselves or even the thief, who knows? I have a constant fear of running out of time and a terror of unfinished business, be it vacuuming, putting boxes in the loft or paying a bill ... it needs to be done when it needs to be done, not later on!

As part of this, 2015 feels like a year for completing unfinished items, jobs, projects, ideas ... call them what you will. Not just those things from the last six years, but those from my lifetime. The thief has left me with the idea that when it is my time to bow out, however and whenever that happens, I will not regret the things that I have not done. So now, my efforts seem heightened with an urgency to meet those financial challenges, have my ambitions in place and unfinished business.

#

I'm socialising a little more. Whilst I still do not manage well in groups, I have made an effort to accept invitations to dinner and smaller gatherings. I make sure that I sit beside someone who I know well and who will help with those missed questions. Of course, when you've been out of the loop for a while, those invitations are few and far between at times, but at least I am now better placed to try to make the most of them when they do come along. However, I'm generally limited to during the day, as by the evening fatigue still has me almost insensible, but I try to make the most of a daytime social life. The only problem with it is that sometimes, the more I regain confidence from this semi-socialising circle I now have, which I am of course so grateful for, the more I also miss what I have lost.

#

My memory remains a big challenge. In this regard I'm truly grateful that I was such an avid photograph album creator. I have relied on these albums for so much information, one for nearly every year of my children's lives or in the early days two years to one album, back in the pre-digital era when we took fewer photos. These photos have kept me in contact with my old self and those around me during a time when a lot of very real contact seemed to be missing, when it was most needed.

Something that saddens me is the lack of contact with most of my brothers; it's now practically non-existent apart from one with whom I've enjoyed a good relationship and sporadic contact with. In reality this hasn't really changed a lot over the years. Although I see some of them when I go to Ireland, they rarely come to see me. Of course, some of them came for my 'wake' (as I truly believed it to be at the time) and this says something. Yet since then it's remained with me to be the one making the effort to see my family, it's the price I pay for moving to a foreign country. Sadly, since Encephalitis I now have less energy and ability for the letter writing and phone calls, and much less so for those which go unacknowledged.

#

I still try to remain positive, whilst bristling inwardly at those who tell me to do so of course. But overall I feel very inadequate at times with regard to my ability to cope with daily life. I try to help my children and help with my grandchildren as much as I can – there are four of them by now, my two children each have two children. But any and all assistance I can offer is within limitations. It still saddens me that I will never hear my grandchildren's voices properly and I often find it very difficult to understand them. They are patient with me, bless them, more so than I am with myself, but then they have never known me any different, which I also feel sad about. They have always known me with hearing problems and incapacities. This is the woman that I am now.

#

There are little things too, smaller, or is that taller changes? I have avoided wearing my ankle length camel coat as since being ill I've been concerned that it dropped on the ground – heels being what's needed but unfortunately something I still can't really do. I had the coat cleaned and periodically I spy it, hanging in my wardrobe with its '09 cleaning tag. Today I put it on, bracing myself for the same problem, particularly as I've been dismayed with recent photographs from my brother, feeling that I look just like an old woman from the hills, so stooped and unsteady looking. To my surprise my coat now comes to my ankles, not to the ground. It seems that even though I'm still without my heels, I have uncurled somewhat.

#

So it seems I am regaining a more 'normal' state. However, the fact remains that I am disabled across all parts of my function but I am not registered disabled, apart from my registration for hearing. This brings perks, of a disabled railcard which includes a companion ticket. Unfortunately though this system is more expensive than the equivalent travel ticket I used to buy …getting a regular last-minute ticket costs less!

#

I've let go of medication now, continuing with my EFT, my acupuncture and herbs. In truth, I've been off all medication for a few years now although this tends to present a misleading situation. When I go for any medical attention there seems to be some surprise that I'm not 'on anything.' But the thing is, it's been proved that medication will not improve any of the issues that I still have; I've persisted but decided, along with the various consultants, that it's a futile exercise to keep taking them. I think too that the consultants recognise and accept that I really don't want to keep taking them when there's so little chance of them making any real difference. The consultants are affable enough and always happy to discharge me with a cheery "you can always come back if you need to …!" I'm grateful to them, but would be more grateful not to have to need them again.

#

Emerging from Encephalitis feels like being a chrysalis or a caterpillar ... there's that breath-held stillness of the unknown, waiting to see what will emerge. Will it be a delicate butterfly, to be glanced at and admired as it sits on some beautiful flower, that's too fragile to touch for fear of doing some damage to its gossamer wings? Or will it be a hairy moth which will be sprayed with a poisonous aerosol or fed camphor so it will not interfere with the pretty things in life, the rich tapestries and finery we surround ourselves with ... all before it has the chance to spread its wings and show itself off in its full glory?

I still don't really know which it will be for me, who my predators and protectors will be. At times I feel so much like the moth: I want to hide inside the wardrobe, away from those who don't acknowledge to me that they are seeing anything different from that old familiar shell that they have always known; those who try to be with me as they always have, with a dismissive "you're doing OK, you'll soon be back to your old self" but never taking the time to look past the old external shell, because the truth is, it's this which remains when both the butterfly and moth have long flown, the shell with the empty insides.

But at the end of the day, the end of this road, I am still me. Even with the ongoing issues that I have to deal with, I'm getting to a place of being able to say that I had a life before Encephalitis, before my affable caterpillar self was shoved, inert into a chrysalis of the Encephalitis kind. I'm now emerging and shrugging off the belief that these last 6 years, with the impact of the thief, was the total of my life. Yes, I know the thief has come and gone, yet will never leave; what's left is another part of the me I have to live with. I started out as someone who was always looking to give back and now, with this Encephalitis experience, my EFT journey and the fact that I can now practice EFT professionally, I am still, although another person in many ways, the same person who can give something back. Thief or no thief, there's still the rest of me.

The Woman I Used To Be

Part I

I'll stay with my daughter
If that's all right, it's safer than staying
Alone for the night.
A few days in bed will rid me of flu, soon I'll be feeling as good as new
Then I'll return to the me I once knew.

No warning came, to tell me why
No phone call, letter or little good bye,
I didn't know that I had to fly-

A company to run, a job to do
A daughter, a son, a new granddaughter too
Daughter in law, son in law, people, things, counselling too -
Where is the 'I' we all knew?

You don't seem yourself, you're confused to me
We'll need to call the GP
But it's out of hours, do you think they'll agree?
Let's try, then wait and see
We need to find who you used to be

The doctor arrives to search for me
Checks and tests, to some degree
"The Prime minister's name, who is he?
The queen, her name too, who is she?"

Push hands, push feet.....
Silly questions......
But it helps to get a picture....
Yes, confused they agree....

Phone calls, arrangements, have to be made
Just to be sure there's a bed, a bag to be packed for an overnight stay
Arriving in hospital to find my bed,
Is where my memory ends.

A medical unit for admissions
No memory of bed, yet I sleep
In some distant trance I wonder, “Will they find the old me”,
The person I used to be?

Young doctors, old doctors, neurologists, nurses
Who come from all over the world?
Even the Draculas to collect my blood-the search has got to be good.
The tap, tap, tapping of the MRI
The lumbar punctures to extract the spinal fluid
Nearly two weeks go by before a result
The decision from all these tests is here
A virus; now which strain could it be?
Encephalitis they agree;
Let treatment commence, then wait and see

They prod and they poke, and I really don’t care
Just wait till they tell me they found me some where
I don’t know my children or baby E or her daddy, who can that man be?
They’re also waiting, praying and prancing
Unaware of their torment, I sleep

Part II

But alas their persecution also finds me
Encased in a horse box all that I see
Are ghouls and ghosts that really scare me
I'm going someplace that I don't want to be,

Ghouls and ghosts hang around me
Large and giggly and white as can be
Floating around waiting to trick me, they want me in a sanatorium you see
This is a place that really scares me.

Will no one believe this is not the real me?
I shriek at the nurse, who won't listen to me
I want my daughter why can't she see,
She is the only one who knows me?

I tell the nurse I am scared of the place that you are sending me to
My daughter will come if I ask her to
"But she will be sleeping now: it's the middle of the night,
But we can call her if we really must"

She duly arrives bless her soul
To sit in the day room till I feel in control
Then she can go,
And let paranoia and hallucinations again take hold,
The horse box is coming, I know in my soul,
To take me where I don't want to go.

Four weeks have passed and I'm getting better
Now it's time for the discharge letter
And then I'll be homeward bound
For a week I remain there and hardly utter a sound!

But all is not well and the ambulance comes,
To take me back where I might be found
For another four weeks, bed bound.

But where is the capable confident me?
No driving or flying, that's not 'she',
I can't go to work, my car's out of bounds
Bundled up and shifted about
Now how am I meant to get around?

My son is gone where he needs to be
He can fly, unlike me!
I'll live with my daughter,
It's safer they say
And go to my house when my son comes to stay.
Will it always have to be this way?

Part III

Discharged
Once more the same words echo
'What now?'
A full recovery you should make
Without a hint of how long it might take

I can't read or write and I feel so alone
But at least for now I can use the phone
Shuffling around, so much out of bounds
Too weak to manage alone

My nerves seem to jangle with fear and dread
Oh! How I wish I was dead!
The baby cries (and so do I)....
It breaks my heart to hear her,
But her silence is worse...
What will cure all the ills my body holds?
I try everything from acupuncture to a Carnelian stone

I pray I won't die, but hope that I do
Better all round if I exit on cue
Not just imprisoned in a house, I'm imprisoned inside of me
Tinnitus comes to plague me,
Prevents me from hearing the things that would help me...

Misunderstanding and rows make an unhappy home
Why can't they see?
How hard it is for me
To be contradicted and corrected constantly,
Fear and suspicion engulf me
Why do they whisper so?

Yet people and pictures tempt me back
To recall and regain my forgotten past...
My room is littered with paper piles
That consume all the things I should know
All covered in yellow post-its
To tell me where they go...

Hospital appointments that never stop
My sight and hearing both going to pot
Deaf now, another shock!
I'm meant to be improving, so why deaf now?
I try to lip-read, but people don't look up when they speak
With a moon face from steroids I feel I look like a freak

I no longer hear baby cry,
Is she breathing or did she die?
I want to check, but that's not my right,
Parents are there for her all through the night...
But I can't stop this fear take flight.

When people come to visit me, we relocate to my own abode
Fear starts all over again-
Will I ever manage alone?
With fear and trepidation I climb the stairs to bed,
But nothing seems to quiet the turmoil in my head

Oh! Why didn't I die?
I'm sure it would have been the easier way
But someone deemed that I should stay
Perhaps I've a debt to pay,
With the punishment that's on the way

Part IV

A stranger now to all I once knew
I slowly scramble to a life anew
"A full recovery you should make"
No compass, clock or calendar to state
Just how near or precisely what date

Home alone the days just go,
Everything takes time because now I'm so slow.
No complaint though from my little godsend
Because of her age she can't comprehend
And accepts me in the beginning as in the end

The sensory team visit, talk endlessly and say
'You'll be registered deaf'
As if that in itself would help.
A pager's supplied to alert me
To smoke and ringing of bells
Though before I get there, their pealing ends.

Social workers arrive; clip board in hand
Giving the notion of the helping hand.
I tell them what I know I need but they pay little heed!
I don't fit in their box, they concede
I'm not in the right band so flexibility be damned

They question entitlement: "Are you worth it?" in other words
The answer always seems the same
With another appointment for more info to gain
Again comes the same old refrain
Wrong box, wrong band!

There's nothing they can do,
But give me a monetary sum,
Then refer my case, not me, to the fairer charges crew.
Into the computer they would plug me
If I agreed with their demand
You can shop on line, buy.....on line
No question of reintegration
T'was dismissed right out of hand.

Then without words -----
You're worth nothing if you can't get up
And walk and do something-----
I feel such a desperate need to talk;
They walk!

Twelve months now passed
No week yet appointment free
Then suddenly I met, my next 'godsend'
Who introduced me to EFT?

For two long years now we've tapped and tapped
And cried and cried, then eventually laughed!
While I grieved for the life that I once knew
The respect and kindness my herbalist prescribed
Now supplied.

No judgment, no anger, no urge to blame!
She steered me through stage after stage,
New appointments with promise, yet to no avail
Hospitals so much further afield
Encompass the terror of underground trains
She was even there when they told me,
I now have to void with a tail!

My daughter and friend see my business through
No reference from them of the fairer charges crew
While I stay off with this little flu!
And just watch.
As my work they do.

If positive thinking could cure all ills
The NHS would have no bills
Three long years and still no end
Discharged from one, another to begin...
My shuffle is better, the pain contained
Efforts confirming how sore and slow

But to my appointments I still have to go!
Lifts, taxies, hospital transport: Oh No!
If only I could do as I did before
"Get your licence back" the neurologist said

"I'm not able to drive" I cry
"Just confidence" he sighs,
And then when I drive, I cry

Maybe all I can do, that no one's yet prescribed,
Is sit back and bide my time
Cease the search for the 'me I used to be'
And find a me that is new to be
Put my trust in the Lord and hope
That he will help to find,
A *ME* that once more shines.

Acknowledgements and Resources

My journey has seen the involvement of so many people, professionally of course as well as family, friends, acquaintances and new people who have come in to my life directly as a result of the Encephalitis, such as Ranjana. Without adding another several thousand words to what is already a long, but abridged version of my journals, I'd like to acknowledge and thank everyone who has been a part of this epic journey. But, just like the speeches of Oscar winners, I do have to pull out a few extra acknowledgements:

For my recovery

My children and their families.
The medics at the Conquest Hospital, St. Leonards On Sea, who did such a good job of keeping me alive.
The therapists and therapies that kept me living, moving towards a semblance of the woman I used to be. These include various local acupuncturists and my herbalist and acupuncturist in London, Dr. Shen.
My counsellor friends Jane and Glenda, and my ceaselessly supportive manager Dave.
My singing group friend, Mary.
My old business and work colleagues, Ron, Lorraine and Pat.
The Encephalitis Society, who can be found at http://www.Encephalitis.info or have a support line number of 01653 699599.

For getting the story of my journey "out there"

Andy, my very long term and not so old friend who offered to type my mish-mash of journals and diaries, even before she had seen my scrawl. Even once she saw them and cringe-worthy graphic quality of my emotional outpourings, she insisted that she would be able to decipher them. So began her journey of driving the 8 to 10 hours from Cornwall to visit and then return with another box of journals. Her diligence, kindness and excellence in making sense of my scribbles resulted in over 115,000 words in electronic documents, just from my journals alone. My poems add another 20,000 words to this total ~ and these are just the journals and poems I passed over; there are many more bits and parts of half-started note books which still lurk in their boxes, my thoughts of the time, my worst time. In the days when death was very much on my radar, I wrote in my journal that if I did not live to finish my book then Andy was my nominee as the best person to finish it, a task she admits she is very pleased not to have to do.

As the time came to share my story, I appeared to be still here and was introduced to Katherine, who took over to knit this raw material of files and folders, in both electronic and ring binder forms, into a coherent pattern, to edit and make sense of a time which still seems senseless to me and to create this end result; my true account of a life during and after Encephalitis.

Ava Easton, from the Encephalitis Society, for supporting my book by kindly pre-reading and offering advice for my chapter *On Encephalitis* and for contributing the foreword to The Thief in the Night.

Books which have inspired me to tell my own story, and which might be useful for those who have suffered Encephalitis or those supporting them, have included:
Out of It by Simon Hattenstone

Emma's Story, written by her parents Ian and Margaret Shaw. It was Margaret herself who told me "write your book for yourself and get someone other than family to edit it." Sage advice, followed with gratitude.

The Man Who Mistook His Wife for a Hat by Oliver Sacks

Forever Today by Deborah Wearing

These books have been recalled by their presence in my home and by careful sleuthing to identify which was which and which held impact for me. I also remember one with a red and yellow cover.

The only non-Encephalitis book I read which I would recommend is Time Out of Mind by Jane Lapotaire, her memoir of her experience of ABI through cerebral haemorrhage. I cried all the way through her story with empathy, sympathy and a real sense that here is someone who knows what I am going through; she knows what this is like.

Finally, I'd just like to say that there isn't really anybody who has not contributed to my recovery so far, in one way or another, whether these be those who helped me, made me happy, sad, angry or distanced themselves from me. In truth, they have all taught me something and left me open to new learning, new opportunities and new people.

www.ingramcontent.com/pod-product-compliance
Lightning Source LLC
Chambersburg PA
CBHW020656270326
41928CB00005B/143
9781783822034